NOT WHAT YOU THINK

*How hypnotherapy (and losing 100 lb.)
changed my mind and my life, and
how it can change yours, too!*

RAY POPE

Clinical & Medical Hypnotherapist

an introduction to Hypnotherapy and its benefits

D1127672

This book is dedicated to my dear wife, Susan, my partner in this incredible journey, and to my children, Daniel (on the left) and Rachel (the bride), who bring me such constant joy and inspire me in ways that they will never really know.

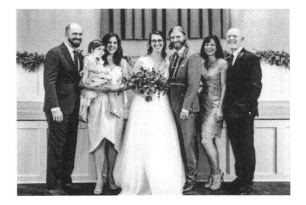

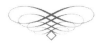

CONTENTS

INTRODUCTION

This book feels more like an organic growth that developed from my interest in hypnotherapy rather than a concerted effort to simply write a book. Can an exercise that took countless hours over months and months still be a surprise?

I did not set out to write a book. It happened like this. I received an invitation to complete an education and certification program from two of the best instructors in the world of hypnotherapy. Classes would not start for another six months or so. I wanted to make the best use of my time before classes began in order to prepare myself for a career in hypnotherapy. With my background in digital marketing, I knew that I needed a plan for launching my practice, and a major component of that plan would be the implementation of a website.

The website would need to include my personal experience with hypnotherapy as a client, a general explanation of hypnosis and hypnotherapy, particularly addressing misconceptions, and an outline of services. As I pondered these elements, I realized that I had the outline to a book. Well, why not write one? The exercise of writing would prepare me for returning to the classroom, at the very least. Whether or not it even saw print, it would offer the material needed for a website, and it would provide a wealth of knowledge about this new field. Committed to the effort, I began writing.

The first complete draft of the content was completed the week before classes began. Since I wrote the book prior to any formal education in hypnosis and hypnotherapy, it has an untrained layman's voice. The classes confirmed that I got most things right – only a few technical changes needed to be made to the original text. The outsider's view and voice remain.

The goal has been to create a tool useful to the understanding of this often misunderstood and mysterious science and to explore what it means practically for individuals, their families, and their friends. Whether you come to the text as a long-time believer in the value of hypnosis in helping people change behaviors, feel better, and perform better, or as a skeptic in the value of such a practice, or as someone in-between, my hope is that a scan of the table of contents will lead you to find something of value – something that may offer hope and change for someone who struggles.

Thank you!

PART 1

UNEXPECTED JOURNEY: CHANGING MINDS ABOUT CHANGING MINDS

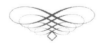

CHAPTER 1

A MATTER OF THE HEART

W e have no evidence of heart issues causing the chest pains, but let's schedule you to see a cardiologist for a stress test to rule out that as a cause."

It seemed like no big deal. I certainly didn't think it was a heart problem. All EKGs, chest x-rays, and blood work seemed to indicate the old ticker was just fine. The blood pressure was always a little high, but I just passed that off as white-coat syndrome.

It had something to do with allergies, I reasoned. I spent my youth outside, running through the woods of Florida barefooted like a wild native – I am, after all, one-sixteenth Creek, thank you very much. I had no allergy issues then, but an adult move to Georgia seemed to trigger chest tightness that corresponded with the onset of spring pollen. Each season seemed to get a little worse, a pattern which allergy sufferers transplanted to Georgia confirmed. At a Johns Creek Chamber of Commerce breakfast, the 'medical minute' sponsored by the Gwinnett Medical Center was presented by an otolaryngologist affiliated with the local hospital. I cornered the ENT at one point and described the tightness in my chest that occurred during the spring, and he promptly stated, "Oh, you have asthma." "Asthma?" I questioned. "Not chronic asthma, but allergy induced asthma." He explained that it is easily treated, and I left feeling a bit better about the "diagnosis."

Being a typical guy, I knew I could manage these symptoms on my own, and I did with some success. I tested different over-the-counter allergy products and muddled through each spring, often checking my allergy app that would tell me when the pollen count would drop to manageable levels. While spring was the worst for my symptoms, occasionally I would have several weeks of discomfort in the fall, but nothing like that of the spring. Each spring, however, seemed to get a little worse.

Eventually, I married and moved to a more rural county in Georgia . . . more pines, more cattle, the new wife's dog, Roxie . . . Spring hit hard that first year. One Friday evening, I told my wife that the pain and the shortness of breath concerned me, and a foreboding weekend lay ahead. She said, "Let's head to the ER."

There, the staff wasted no time performing all the standard tests associated with chest pains: an EKG and an x-ray. Nothing there of any concern. The doctor accepted my self-diagnosis of allergy-induced asthma and ordered a breathing treatment. Ah, immediate relief! I felt relieved and headed home with a prescription for allergy medicines, an inhaler, and a note to follow up with my primary care doctor.

Several weeks later, I sat with my doctor, and we discussed the results of my now second EKG and blood work. Again, nothing of interest appeared so the doctor sent me home with Singulaire, and orders to keep the inhaler handy. "Oh, by the way," he added, "let's give you some nitroglycerin capsules, just in case it turns out that it's something else." Prophetic words.

Everything should have been under control.

Except that it wasn't.

All of my adult life, even though I was overweight, I hit the gym religiously. Cardio was always part of my regular routine. The cardio was the reason why my heart was in such good shape, right? But now, as I was coming off the medical visits. I began to notice some changes. Whether I was on the treadmill or the elliptical, after about two minutes, I began to feel chest pain. Was it my lungs? Esophagus? Something else? At first I would simply push through the pain, but it progressively got worse, and I would have to stop. The inhaler seemed to bring immediate relief, but it would not prevent the pain, even if I used it before exercising. The pain could not be exercise-induced asthma, as my doctor had suggested. So, I headed back to the doctor.

I sat facing the doctor. Was he frustrated? Or was he beginning to suspect something more? "Let's get you to a cardiologist and get a stress test. Let's eliminate any heart issues."

I found myself sitting in yet another doctor's office for an interview and yet another EKG, my third one so far. Again, nothing serious enough to cause any concern. The doctor scheduled me for a stress test within the next ten days, and I headed home to wait things out. I had no great expectation that the stress test would reveal anything; it was just another medical procedure to endure.

On the day of the test, another cardiologist performed the procedure, injecting the dye into my veins. The doctor and I talked about my recent medical history, and I explained that allergies were most likely my problem. I also told him that I expected some pain shortly after we would begin the work on the treadmill, and I was correct. The pain came quickly. So did the doctor's diagnosis. I'll never forget his look, almost like a detective gleefully solving a mystery in a gruesome case. He simply stated (did I detect a smile?), "Well, it's not allergies." He then asked if I had taken a small dosage of aspirin that morning, and he gave me a nitroglycerin tablet to take immediately. This was not looking good.

The cardiologist really looked concerned. He wanted to transport me to the hospital across the street to await a prompt heart catheterization. The hospital, however, was full, and no bed was available. With a stern warning to relax and do absolutely nothing, he sent me home to return first thing the next morning for the heart catheterization. There may have been allergy issues, but events had certainly taken a decidedly serious turn.

The next morning, my wife and I arose early and headed to the hospital. I was prepped and moved into the cardiac catheterization lab, where dye and a small camera were inserted into a strategic artery at my hip. As my cardiologist worked, I remained alert, although I really had no sense of what was going on around me. It was apparent, however, that the doctor was a bit frustrated. Catheterizations, optimally, can not only help to find problems, but also to help repair them. For example, if a doctor finds a blockage, he could use techniques to open the passage again.

In my case, the doctor found blockages, four of them. One in particular, probably the main cause of my chest pain, was the left anterior descending artery (or LAD), a branch of the left coronary artery. Because this artery provides blood flow to such a large portion of the body, and blockages there are so dangerous, it is known as the "Widowmaker." My blockage was situated at the intersection of the branching of the left coronary artery, so a simple angioplasty could not be performed without taking on considerable coronary risks.

To fix my problem, doctors would to go in manually and perform open heart surgery. I would not be going home again for a while.

CHAPTER 2

AN OPEN HEART

My destination was the Medical College of Georgia Hospital. After six painful hours lying on a hospital gurney at Doctor's Hospital (one must remain flat and still after catheterizations because doctors do not want to see patients bleed out of the artery they used), I got my first ambulance ride ever. I was unimpressed. The back of a dump truck would have been just as comfortable.

Dr. Dominic Gallo, my cardiothoracic surgeon, came by and introduced himself to me before my transport. He was a confident, gum chewing, former Army surgeon, and he immediately instilled confidence in me. But he was also the first of several to review the risks of what I was about to experience. Surgery would be at 7:30 the next morning.

Events moved along quickly on the eve of my surgery. Nurses and staff began the pre-operation preparation with yet more x-rays and EKGs. In addition, nurses and doctors counseled me on what to expect, both during and after surgery. I was most interested in any potential psychological changes that I might experience beyond the typical challenges of surgery and extended recovery. Would I need some individual counseling? Isn't the heart the center of life and more than a blood pump?

My daughter had made her way to Georgia from Knoxville, Tennessee, where she taught. I was grateful to see her. She has always held tough for her dad, but I could see her concern. My son would be flying in from Texas, where he was attending law school. He would see me after the surgery. Facing the seriousness of open heart surgery, my daughter and I developed a living will in order to prepare for the worst. Fortunately, we share a love for all things Seinfeld, and those references to Kramer's hilarious living will scene helped to reduce the intensity of the situation.

As people moved out and preparations finished up, I had time to ponder what lay ahead. My nurse offered me a mild anti-anxiety medication, and I accepted. Peace about the situation came, and I silently prayed. God answered with the peaceful reminder of His sovereignty over all my affairs and that come tomorrow I would continue to serve Him, either in this life or the next. The apostle Paul had it right in Philippians 1:21. I slept well.

Bright and early on July 13, 2016, nurses woke me and prepared me for surgery. The first item of business, was a full body shave from head to toe. FULL body. Then off to the surgical suite to prepare for a 7:30 a.m. call with the surgeon.

Since the development of heart transplants and other advanced heart-related surgeries is so common today, I never asked for details regarding the actual surgical procedure. I simply kept myself from thinking about what was about to happen to me, my body. The team made sure to explain the surgical events, however. First, I would be anesthetized. Then, my body would be packed in ice to bring my blood pressure and organ activity down. My chest would be cut open. First the skin, and then the sternum would be sawn through. (Today, I carry an eight inch vertical reminder down the middle of my chest.) My breast bone and ribs would be pulled apart by about five inches, leaving a forty square inch hole in my chest.

Next, another human being would reach into that cavity and take my beating heart into his hands and then strategically cut my life-sustaining arteries and attach them to a heart-lung machine that would make life possible while my "plumbing" was rearranged. Good vessels would be clipped from my leg and grafted into those arteries, bypassing the blockages. One key bypass was called a LIMA graft, a procedure that takes the Left Internal Mammary Artery and redirects it to the LAD artery, attaching it below the blockage. If the body were a map, the surgeon is, in effect, taking a major thoroughfare heading north, cutting it, moving it down the front of the heart, and

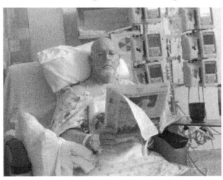

"merging" it with a super highway heading south. Incredible! And that is just one of the grafts.

Fortunately, I have no memory beyond the pre-op room. My earliest memory after the surgery was a foggy look around the recovery room. I was still intubated but I do remember clearly seeing my daughter next to me. She relates how I awakened later in a good humor, wondering if anyone had seen the truck that had hit me.

I spent the next few days in the CICU – Cardiac Intensive Care Unit. There I learned that I was a "cabbage," the name given to patients who had received coronary artery bypass grafts. The stay in the CICU introduced me to what was going to be a very long road back. I realized, again, maybe at an even deeper level, how sick the professionals really thought I had been, as well as the limits to my mortality.

The biggest concern post-surgery was a continuing problem with atrial fibulation or A Fib. I was told it was a relatively common problem occurring in about fifty percent of heart surgery patients. It was a temporary problem with most patients. Unfortunately, it became a significant issue for me for a while. Wires had been attached to my heart and ran out through my chest for this very reason. Doctors would run power through these wires in an effort to restore sinus rhythm. These efforts were unsuccessful.

Since I was at a teaching hospital, I became a source of educational attention as medical students and others paid me visits. On one occasion, a doctor and his entourage approached me and began another procedure. This one entailed shocking the heart back into rhythm. In order to do so, they first administered an LSD-type hallucinogen, which had me seeing and hearing things I hope never to experience again!

My heart returned to normal sinus rhythm on and off, but the staff ultimately determined that I was well enough to return home. The A Fib occurred only one other time after I returned home. I sympathize with anyone who suffers with A Fib regularly; it is a very oddly uncomfortable feeling.

Although I was very sick, it was in the CICU that I realized how much better off I was than others around me. Nurses gathered me up to walk me around the halls two days after surgery, and I caught glimpses of my CICU neighbors. As I passed the rooms – all with glass walls to allow regular monitoring – I observed very sick, very out-of-shape patients. I resolved then that I would get into better shape after all this was over!

Finally I was released to go home. My son spent the last night with me in the hospital. Nurses pushed my wheelchair to the front of the hospital while my wife pulled the car around. My first instructions: sit in the back seat. Because my chest had been pieced back together, an airbag deployment in a wreck could have very serious repercussions. I was fine in the back seat, clutching a pillow to my chest. Medical staff recommend using a small pillow throughout the day to enable adequate coughing and alleviate the discomfort. It would be months before I did not regularly hold a pillow to my chest, particularly when I slept.

Although the doctors assured me that my heart and circulatory system were operating well, my body felt broken. I walked like an old man, slowly and gingerly. I could never quite get comfortable. A sneeze or a cough was enough to cause mild panic, and I would grasp my small chest pillow and hold on for dear life. I was, however, determined to recover from this trauma.

I worked from home, so getting to work would not be too much trouble. Within a week, I was back in the office, firing up the computer and checking on my clients. Looking back, I see how amazingly blessed I was to be able to stay on top of work as well as I did.

Two weeks after surgery, I ventured out for worship. Fellow congregants were amazed. I suppose my years in the gym had, even with my excess weight, benefitted my body. At a follow up visit to the surgeon, I met a fellow alumnus from the CICU. He was still looking peaked and using a walker to get around. He and his family were surprised to see me walking in looking, dare I say, normal. The doctor was pleased with my progress, as well. That would be the last time I would see him.

Although I was healing insanely well, my body still had much rehabilitation to endure. Home health care nurses and physical therapists made regular visits. We set short goals: walk to the end of the driveway, walk up the street and back, walk half a block, walk a block . . . Progress was in the small steps. One of my greatest blessings was in the back yard: the swimming pool. The buoyancy of the water in addition to the summer sunshine provided such a great relief to my post-surgery aches and pains. I began by simply cruising around the pool on a float, but later I straddled a pool noodle and used my legs and arms to "swim" laps.

My body was healing and I was feeling better, but I was still heavily medicated. I weaned myself off the narcotics for pain as quickly as I could. I came off the blood thinner I had been prescribed to help offset the A-Fib within a month's time. With the surgery, my blood pressure had improved, but I was still on blood pressure medication, a miserable drug for my poor body. One Sunday morning, I neglected to take it in the rush to get out the door. It took me a while to determine why I felt so much better that morning! The world was so much clearer! I was elated to get off that particular one for good after several months.

The one medication that would become a real battle was the statin. I suppose my body chemistry makes me overly sensitive to these medications. At the onset, the statin turned me into an old man, making my body ache and my moods swing. Unfortunately for me, the 'standard of care' for patients who have undergone coronary bypass surgery calls for the use of statins. Get used to it, Ray.

Life had really taken on a different feeling after surgery. A friend of mine who appeared to be the picture of health had suffered a heart attack in his early fifties. After that, I could never look at him without thinking, "It's only a matter of time." Now, I viewed myself that same way. Any delusions of invincibility were gone. I was indeed a mortal man.

Even though my days seemed numbered now, I wanted to make the best of them. I needed to take pressure off my heart and circulatory system. I needed to clean up the blood flowing through my veins. My weight remained the same, although most bypass patients lose fifteen to twenty percent of their body weight during the process of the surgery and recovery. Not me. I didn't make quite ten percent. I had been a fat kid growing up – before being a fat kid was the norm. I "shot up" in high school and became "large normal" for a while, and I had lost substantial weight several times in my life. For a period of thirteen years in my twenties and thirties I had been an active runner, and my weight remained average through that exercise. Since then, however, I had blossomed to the 'big bone,' 'husky,' and 'stout' categories. I suppose I had achieved a peace with my being 'heavy.'

I needed to change. Now. I never wanted to go through anything like open-heart surgery again. I wanted to feel better.

I needed to get off these awful medications. I wanted to see my children married, and I wanted to enjoy my grandkids. I needed time with my wife. I needed to lose weight!

My first efforts, post-surgery, proved futile. Feeling better simply made food taste that much better. As I improved physically, I hit the gym, but in my mind, that just meant that I deserved more food! And my diet was nowhere as "clean" as it needed to be.

Lord, I needed to make some changes!

CHAPTER 3

FROM A SERIOUS SKEPTIC . . .

Months passed after surgery, and while I had been able to maintain my business, I had not been able to grow it very much. My wife and I decided it was time to focus more on re-establishing my business foothold in the Atlanta area. Our target was to work through three chambers of commerce, one of which I was already actively working with. I would spend a great deal of time on the road, but we felt the approach was worth the effort.

All three chambers offered weekly networking meetings. At all of the meetings, business people meet other business people to share what they do in a variety of ways, including brief elevator speeches. Through such networking, we help each other to market and grow our businesses. One fun activity at these chamber meetings is to share door prizes, gifts from each business where winners are drawn from a hat full of business cards.

My business, a one-man job, was an online marking consulting business that served local businesses and professionals, providing SEO (search engine optimization) work along with reputation marketing and management services. Tag lines are important for name recognition, and I had fine-tuned mine: "Why talk to the priest when the Pope's in town? Ray Pope, Atlanta Inbound."

Years earlier I had witnessed a fellow who weekly gave away a jar of jelly beans. It had become a popular prize, as well as quite the tradition at that particular chamber. Everyone wanted the 'honor' of winning it. I was active in only one chamber at that time, Johns Creek, and the number of door prize offerings had dwindled a bit. As I was walking through a Kroger one day, I saw bottles of Sweet Baby Ray's barbeque sauce. Aha! I bought a bottle – about $3.00 – created my own little logo that said "Atlanta Inbound brings the sauce" and taped it to the bottle. Voila! My own personal door prize!

I never meant for it to be a long term giveaway, just a fun one-time thing. However, it turned into a hit with the members there. I repeated it, and then someone pointed out that door prizes had to meet a $10 minimum. He was correct, and I did not mind stopping the practice; it had all been just for fun anyway. Yet, when I stopped, others asked what had happened to my sauce. Word came down from the 'authorities' that Sweet Baby Ray's would be an exception to the ten dollar rule. Maybe people enjoyed winning it?

As weeks went along, I decided to leverage the barbeque sauce a little more. After meetings. I would ask the winner to pose for a photo holding the sauce. They would hold it like they had won an Oscar, and I would post the picture on my business Facebook page and on LinkdIn, offering a plug for the business and contact information. It was a lot of fun.

Networking meetings held by the chambers were open to just about any business. Chamber membership is not required, but non-members pay an attendance fee. As a result, all kinds of businesses attend, occasionally even people seeking work. Some may be start-ups, a few are muti-level marketing ventures, and others defy any real label. I once sat between two "healers." I'm still not sure what they actually did.

One profession represented at the meetings always "creeped me out" a bit: hypnotherapy. I have heard from others that they have the same reaction. Maybe those therapists scared us: "Don't let them look you in the eye!" I always found some way to look away. I did not want them to see my professional revulsion, so I would look at the floor, at the wall, anywhere but in the eyes. I put them in the same category as TV faith healers – of the devil they were!

Your reaction may be the same as mine had been. In my case, a number of experiences had contributed to my limited understanding of hypnosis. I had seen the "cluck like a chicken" stage shows that had been an embarrassment to its participants. Who on earth would give up his own personality to a stranger? I had also seen Woody Harrelson in the movie *Now You See Me*. Could someone really be hypnotized that quickly and controlled so completely? I was not about to find out! I knew also that there were athletes, such as professional golfers, who had used hypnotherapy. I did not consider such use cheating, and I could not blame them since so much money lay on the line. But I could not escape the idea that such practice was a form of pseudoscience, a dark practice with no real merit.

As for me, a fellow with strong Christian convictions, there was a tendency to lump hypnotherapists in with fake prophets, soothsayers, astrologists, and other demonic agents. I had never really done a thorough Biblical analysis of hypnosis and hypnotherapy, but I trusted my gut. [What I know now makes all the difference in the world. I deal with these and many other myths and misconceptions about hypnosis and hypnotherapy in CHAPTER 13.]

Eventually, one of "them" (hypnotherapists) won the Sweet Baby Ray's sauce at the Johns Creek Chamber during Wednesday morning networking. I knew him only casually, and he seemed a nice enough guy. He dressed sharply, spoke intelligently, and seemed friendly enough, but I knew what he did…although I later discovered that I really knew nothing! But winners always get their photos taken with me. So after the meeting adjourned, I made my way to meet Ken Thompson. When I walked up to him, I did not see the barbeque sauce. "I gave it away," he explained. Ken saw my expression. "My wife and I don't use barbeque sauce." My expression must have demanded further explanation. "You see, she went from a size 14 to a size 4, and I lost 75 pounds. That's why we both decided to become hypnotherapists."

Now he had my attention. So this lean, trim man had been as bad off as I was now? He and his wife had both successfully lost weight using hypnotherapy and had kept the weight off. Obviously they had changed their eating habits, and the barbeque sauce loaded with sugar and calories was not on their diet. On top of all that, they had pursued this profession.

At this point my mind began to race. I needed and wanted to lose weight. I needed to make some life changes to avoid going through what I had just gone through. I had attempted diet changes and worked out regularly, but I knew down deep that the same habit remained locked inside. My yo-yo dieting could not be good for my health. So I lobbed a tough question at him: "Like, you can make me like broccoli?"

I really despised broccoli. Like Newman on Seinfeld, I considered it a "vile weed," a smelly, unappetizing vegetable not fit for man nor beast. Of course, I had a long list of foods I avoided, most of which were vegetables. I had a saying that I did not like anything that was good for me, and I loved all foods that were bad for me. I did not eat tomatoes (unless they were crushed up and loaded with sugar in ketchup or in pizza sauce), Brussel sprouts, cauliflower, and so much more. When I ate, I ate entirely too much. What I ate was loaded with sugars, carbs, and fats. If he could have me eating broccoli, I knew I had a chance at change.

"Sure, no problem," was how I interpreted his look. (He was a man of his word. In a matter of weeks, I would devour broccoli and other wonderful tasting vegetables, asking for more! But I get ahead of myself...)

"So, you do that with hypnosis?"

"Yes, hypnosis is part of it."

Hmmmm. He sounded pretty confident. Maybe I'm too cerebral to be hypnotized. "I've never been hypnotized. I'm not sure that would actually work on me."

Rather than respond directly to my comment, he defined the idea of hypnosis. "Have you ever been driving on the highway, lost in thought thinking about work, and thirty minutes later you realize you have not been paying attention to your driving? That's a form of hypnosis you do to yourself. The subconscious operates in fascinating ways. A lot of our most serious decisions are made there. If you can get lost in a book or a TV show, or if you daydream, you can be hypnotized. Come by for a consultation, on the house, and we'll go into more detail."

Dang! It did make sense. Maybe this was the answer. Maybe I should give it a try. What would people think? Well, they just would not know; it would be my little secret.

He had me, and it would be one of the best decisions I ever made for myself in my life.

I took him up on his offer of a complimentary session. And then I signed up full time.

It did not take me long to realize that Ken knew his field and that the field was more science than hocus-pocus. I developed a high level of trust in him and his work. There was a cost, of course, since he is a professional and every working man is worth his wages. But I knew that this work was an investment in myself, and that I was worth it.

It would take me a few short weeks to grasp the basics involved with my therapy. One thing that did make sense to me was the use of relaxation techniques in combination with repetition, much like one would use in perfecting a golf swing. As I explain in greater detail later, the relaxation is not for recovering from fatigue, but it is the first step in creating a particular state of mind, a state of mind that does not learn or change, like our active, conscious mind. This particular state of mind is oh so valuable in controlling our habits, instincts, and drives. The repetition gives our minds the opportunity to dislodge unfavorable behaviors and replace them with new ones, the new behaviors that clients, not the therapist, select and direct.

The most fascinating part for me was the control that I gained over myself throughout the process. I expected a sense of vulnerability during the therapy sessions, but that was not the case at all. For the longest time, I thought that the hypnosis itself was not really working because I always felt in control and aware. I did not become unconscious or feel like I was "out of it" at all. In fact, though relaxed, I was never more zeroed-in on what was happening.

I also appreciated the fact that my targeted goal was not some cookie-cutter approach to weight loss. Throughout the whole process, we repeatedly worked on my issues, my needs, my desires, and my objectives. (The nuts and bolts of hypnotherapy for weight loss are explained in detail in Part III.)

Everything was so different than what I had expected. Only one big, weighty issue remained . . . would it work?

CHAPTER 4

. . . TO BELIEVER

I t worked! I really lost weight, but I lost so much more!

I had come in with a poor overall daily diet. I loved cheese and crackers, carbs of any kind, coffee loaded with creamer, sweets, diet cokes, pizzas... well, you get the point. I did not appreciate the choices that a healthy diet offered. Looking back, I see how quickly the changes in me took place.

The dreaded broccoli became a favorite in a matter of weeks. How hypnotherapy works is hard to comprehend. Even as I progressed through the therapy, I was unsure how the process actually worked. I felt no big changes, but ever so subtly my desires began to change. I wanted to taste new foods just for fun for the first time in my life. Broccoli, cauliflower, brussel sprouts, spinach, and other greens began to grace my plate. Tomatoes even! How did this change happen? What caused the switch to flip in my desires? These were lifetime, ingrained habits and feelings, and suddenly I was enjoying clean, healthy foods! One side benefit to eating cleanly is that my sense of taste heightened. I loved experiencing all the new flavors.

Cleansing my palate involved more than simply eating the right foods. One accomplishment of my therapy was establishing aversions to the foods that I needed to avoid. With some foods, like pizza and fried chicken, I began to sense the heavy greasiness of the foods. The more I thought about the grease and fat in these foods, the more revulsion I felt toward them.

In other situations, recognition that these foods were poison to me created the aversion. Foods full of carbohydrates, sugars, and preservatives became less and less appealing. I was surprised at the speed with which I could abandon diet soft drinks, a real addiction for me. I knew all the scientific studies showed the danger of such drinks, but it was the hypnotherapy that gave me the tools to act upon that knowledge.

With each session, the hypnotherapy made more and more sense. The diet at the heart of the process generated serious weight loss, and the combination of good, clean food and caloric limitations paid off right away and throughout the whole process.

I began my journey at the beginning of March weighing about 270 pounds, a solid weight for my 5'11" frame. Almost fifteen years earlier I had dropped to just under 220 pounds, so I thought that 220 pounds would be the best that I could reasonably expect. Ken, however, believed we needed to aim for a greater decrease. In my running days during my thirties, I managed to keep my weight in the 180s, but I could not imagine getting there again. However, with Ken's encouragement, we set a goal to lose eighty pounds.

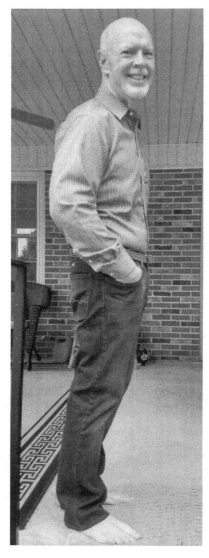

A couple of months later in May, my son graduated from law school, and I showed up forty pounds lighter. By the time my birthday rolled around in August, I had almost reached our original goal of eighty pounds. After reading BMI charts that indicated I was at the heavy end of average, I determined to lose still more. I steadily dropped to below 200 pounds, a huge benchmark in my progress.

Ken encouraged me to aim for 90 pounds, so I kept losing, right on through the Thanksgiving and Christmas holidays. I reached my goal of 90 pounds by the first of the year. It was now time to "re-feed," adding in a variety of foods and upping my caloric intake. As I did, however, a phenomena happened...I continued to lose weight! By the end of February, I had lost 100 pounds.

Some people would be thrilled to get down to their college weight or high school weight. I had managed to hit my middle school weight, a weight that I carried when I was a foot shorter.

As a heavy adult, certain numbers depressed me, so I

avoided them. Now, however, those same numbers amazed me. I dropped from a solid forty-four inch waist to a thirty-two waist, a size I probably had not seen since elementary school! My coat size dropped from a fifty to a forty. My shirt size dropped from a 17 1/2 to a 15. My shoe sized dropped from an eleven to a ten and a half, and even my hat size dropped considerably. I had to replace my entire wardrobe!

But wait! There's more! My overall health had corresponding improvements. My blood pressure, a perpetual battle for me, dropped to normal readings (and sometimes below normal). My BMI, or Body Mass Index, hit 15.5 (a slightly underweight measurement). My oxygen counts, blood sugar count, and cholesterol levels all indicated I was a normal, healthy man. My doctor shook his head in disbelief. He continued to reduce my statin medication until I was on the lowest dosage possible. I finally removed myself from them altogether because they gave me such fits with side effects. Without them, my numbers stayed normal, so I opted to feel better without them.

My body now feels like that of a teenager, and I move freely and easily. I enjoy the energy I have, without the naps I needed in the past. Every minute of every day gets better. At the gym, I continue to make gains I never thought possible. I can now muscle through one hundred unassisted dips (10 sets of 10), whereas before the weight loss, I required a 120 pound counterbalance to complete only one.

At my last session of diet hypnotherapy, Ken complimented me on my success and my diligence during the process. And then he floated an idea . . .

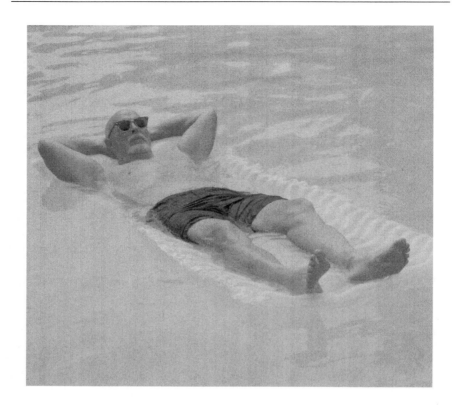

CHAPTER 5

. . . TO PRACTITIONER AND ADVOCATE

Hypnotherapy intrigued me. As a converted skeptic, maybe I had a tendency to over-embrace my new discovery. Ken and his wife, Lisa, had a fascinating story to tell. Their love for helping people improve their lives was evident, and they truly embraced their profession.

Others had noticed my obvious weight loss and had consulted with Ken, as well. They had all succeeded with their goals, and they simply glowed with their weight loss. Others had consulted with Ken for sleep issues and had reported immediate and life changing results. Although I had not seriously formulated a career change, I suppose I was slowly being rerouted toward that direction.

At my last session, Ken spoke about getting to know me through our therapy process, but we had also continued to interact through our weekly business networking activities. He asked me if I had ever considered being a hypnotherapist; he thought I'd make a good one. He let me know that such recommendations were rare from him but that he felt confident in my skills. We discussed the possibility a bit more. I had questions, and I would have many more over the next few weeks. I am sure that I became a bit of a pest to Ken as I wrestled with the idea, but he always remained good-natured and amiable throughout my barrage of questions.

Ken's career into hypnotherapy had come through Dr. Bob Crow and Dr. Inga Chamberlain, co-directors of Atlanta Center for Hypnosis Training, one the of the nation's most elite and highly regarded hands-on training programs. This program had two sets of classes each year and admitted a very limited number of students. The next sessions were already full, so if I wanted to make this change, I would have to wait six months before beginning my training. I learned that their training program was certified, both by the National Guild of Hypnotists and the American Council of Hypnotist Examiners. Students progress through different levels of certifications, first becoming certified hypnotherapists, then certified clinical hypnotherapists, and ultimately certified clinical and medical hypnotherapists.

As part of my decision-making process, I took Ken's advice and set up an appointment to talk personally with Dr. Crow. I was somewhat familiar with him since Ken had used several brief videos by Dr. Crow early in my weight loss therapy. I scheduled a meeting with Dr. Crow, and he sent me some forms to complete. I thought that I was going to be evaluating Dr. Crow and his program. I did not realize, however, that I would be the one evaluated and interviewed for one of only six spaces available in the fall program.

My interview with Dr. Crow inspired and fascinated me.

The PhD after his name stood for not one, but two degrees from Emory University: one in Behavioral Sciences and the other in Psychology. He had taught classes for the Emory Medical School, and he stated that he sat in on all the medical school classes at least twice. As if I were not impressed already with his "life" credentials before hypnotherapy, he told me that he had worked at the White House as a speech writer for Ronald Reagan. The man had some real life experiences.

During our hour or so together, Dr. Crow made sure to give me a comprehensive look at what I would be experiencing. He took me on a tour of the facilities, explained the educational process I would go through, and showed me video clips of a recent class. I was pleasantly surprised to learn that three prior graduates from his class were practicing medical doctors.

Dr. Crow accepted me into his course, and I accepted the challenge, even though courses would begin in the fall – during football season. (I knew that I was serious when I was willing to sacrifice some of my football time!) Further confirmation that I had made the right choice came when Dr. Crow and I shared a table during a business engagement. After observing me engaging with others during the event, he told me that I would make a superb hypnotherapist. I could only pray that his prophecy would come to fruition.

I was excited – and nervous – and interested. Not one to sit idly by awaiting the start of my new career, I delved deeper into the science and profession of hypnotherapy. My excitement for learning more and for helping others grew. I saw the immense good that I could accomplish, one person at a time, with the tools offered in hypnotherapy. It was during this time that the idea of writing a book that told my story began to germinate. I could deliver, in mostly layman's terms, the story, process, and mission of hypnotherapy to a world very ready for it.

The three stages of the program would be intense and challenging, but very practical. I would have plenty of actual clinical practice and preparation. I completed all the course work, received all the certificates, and left confident in my skills. It was time to start helping people. I opened my practice on the north side of Atlanta with the simple message, "Together, let's make your every day better!"

PART 2

MIDDLE MIND MECHANICS: HYPNOSIS AND HYPNOTHERAPY

CHAPTER 6

IT'S ALL IN YOUR MIND, BUT WHERE?

We live in possibly the most materialistic time in the history of the human race. That is not to say that this particular time is a greater time of selfish desire for "things," however. What I mean by materialism is the idea that unless we see, hear, touch, or sense something, it does not exist, or at least it is not important. This idea, introduced to us mainly during the Age of Enlightenment, crept into nearly all disciplines by the end of the eighteenth century. In such thinking, if we cannot sense it, then we dismiss it, ignore it, laugh at it, insult it. It has made atheism its religion and practical science its idol. It relegates anything beyond the five senses to the mystical, the ghostly, the spiritual, or the ignorant. Such materialism claims a superior intellect. It says, "I don't want to think about those unseen experiences/activities. I am above all of that balderdash." Maybe people who think that way are simply afraid of what they do not know.

The story is told of a man who goes down to the river to read a book. Whilst reading, he notices an old fellow trout fishing. As the fisherman pulls in fish after fish, the man notices a strange behavior. After reeling in a big fish, he tosses it back into the river. After he reels in a small fish, he drops it into a basket, presumably for the night's dinner. Observing the behavior for a while, the observer could no longer contain his curiosity. He dropped his book on the bench, got up, and approached the man. "Pardon me, sir, but I have a question. I observe that as you catch the trout, you save the small ones but toss the large ones. Is there, perhaps, a difference in the flavor?" The fisherman replied, "Oh no, it's not that at all. It's just that I only have a six inch frying pan."

Like the fisherman, it is our tendency to reject ideas that do not fit our preconceived ideas, ideas we do not understand, or ideas we have not yet learned about. Those forces beyond our senses may confuse us or even scare us as they cause us to acknowledge forces beyond ourselves. At best, we raise our eyebrows and simply ignore those ideas which are "beyond us," maybe even relegating them to comedy. At worst, we assume that some concept which does not fit into our "frying pan" must be unwholesome or evil. Maybe as we mature, we simply learn to avoid those things which we do not understand as a form of self-protection. Whatever the case, we miss out.

Hypnosis is one field that is often relegated to the spiritual, the ghostly, or the demonic world, thanks in large part to Hollywood (think *The Manchurian Candidate*). We file hypnosis with Ouija Boards, psychics, palm readers, tarot cards, astrologers, and TV faith healers. When a hypnotist or hypnotherapist stands to speak, we vaguely hear the theme song from *The Twilight Zone* begin to play in our heads.

I want to offset these negative perceptions of hypnotherapy. In Part II of this book, therefore, I will establish the scientific and practical applications of hypnosis as a tool for therapy in offering fast relief for many long term behavioral-related maladies. I want to show that despite our fears or our misgivings, hypnotherapy is actually a tool we all use daily in one form or another. It is how we cope every day. It is how we function every day. It is how we entertain ourselves every day.

Think back to the last time you sat bored at a meeting or in a classroom, for example. What did you do? I would suspect that you daydreamed your way through that tiresome meeting. Daydreaming is actually a form of self-hypnosis!

Or think back to a time you took a long, familiar drive somewhere. Did you suddenly realize that you had not been paying attention to traffic, but rather you had been lost in thought for miles and miles? Although we may be concerned about our inattention, we also know something within us would have reacted to bring us quickly back to reality in a traffic crisis. Such an experience is highway hypnosis.

Or consider the last time you became engrossed in a good book, movie, or football game. In moments like these, time stops and outside distractions disappear. We become hyper-focused and immersed in our experience. Athletes refer to this experience as being "In the Zone." The stereotypical football widow knows this experience all too well. She cannot get her husband's attention at all while his team is battling on the gridiron. It's almost like he is hypnotized! Guess what? He is! Hypnosis is a part of our everyday experiences.

As human beings, we have seen instances in which our instincts or drives take over when we have no real time to think. Sometimes these habits or instincts even trump what we consider appropriate behavior. At times, we may say we did something unconsciously, and we would be exactly correct. We are not just turning a phrase; we are speaking true science.

Where do these experiences exist? How do they function? Is there a way to examine and change the "unconscious" programs that affect us throughout each day in order to improve our lives? We can find the answers in what I call "the Middle Mind."

CHAPTER 7

THE MIDDLE MIND

J.R.R. Tolkien gave us Middle Earth in his *Lord of the Ring* series. With apologies to Tolkien, I now present you with the Middle Mind. This term is in no sense scientific or technical, but just as Tolkien gave us a specific place in which he placed events, I hope to create a metaphorical location to help us build on our understanding of how hypnotherapy works, making more concrete an idea that many consider mysterious.

We are most familiar with the terms *subconscious* or *unconscious* to describe that place between our conscious actions and our unconscious states. Ever since Sigmund Freud defined it, our "subconscious" has become a subject of study from both the scientific and the less-than-scientific communities. Such terms, however, seem to suggest an inaccessibility or otherness that at best leaves us confused, and at worst makes us roll our eyes or feel our skin crawl.

Let us first locate the Middle Mind. Think of brain activity being a path with two somewhat familiar places at each end.

At one end of the path is the mental state of deep sleep, a place we understand as a restful solitude. At the other end of the path is that state of intense, often frenetic activity in which we are wide awake and super alert. Think of this state as a form of alertness we have when we sense danger.

The Middle Mind is that place along the path centered somewhere beyond the normal alertness and light sleep. Historically, the Middle Mind has been referred to as the *unconscious*. Hypnotherapists tend to prefer the term *subconscious* for the same reason that I coined the term Middle Mind: there is a sense that an "un" conscious is a nonentity. For the same reason, I fear "sub"conscious may not move us sufficiently away from the realm of the unknown-known, where we tend to lump all things into either "I get it/see it/feel it" or "I don't get it/it's beyond me." We now know that the unconscious or the subconscious is a very real place, a confirmed state of mind, every bit as real, as functional, and as identifiable as our non-thinking deep sleep and hyper-focused alertness are.

One historical stumbling block to people's understanding of hypnotherapy is the word *hypnosis* itself. Derived from Hypnos, the Greek god of sleep, the term *hypnosis* suggests being in a state of sleep. Now, with both scientific tools of measurement and with personal experiences, we know that a person who is hypnotized still has a very functioning mind, despite being very relaxed. Brain wave activity is quite different in a person sleeping from a person under hypnosis. Brain wave scans actually demonstrate that a person under hypnosis is hyper-aware of what is happening around him and is very much in control of his world.

So, if the mind is not asleep during hypnosis, isn't the Middle Mind the same as the conscious mind? No. The Middle Mind and the conscious mind have two different functions with different operating systems, somewhat like Apple computers running differently from the operating system of a PC. The operating system of the conscious mind thinks logically and sequentially. Its programming language is quantitative and uses words and numbers. The operating system of the Middle Mind works far differently, using abstract, non-sequential thinking. The programming of the Middle Mind is accomplished with images, intuition, feelings, memories, and dreams.

Because of these very different operating systems, programming the Middle Mind cannot be accomplished using the tools of the conscious mind. The two parts do not communicate well. In a sense, parts of the conscious mind can access the Middle Mind, such as the hypnotherapist's words, but once there, those parts are changed and manipulated by the Middle Mind.

The functions of the Middle Mind and the conscious mind are far different, as well. The conscious mind handles alert, thinking activities. When you are at work, carrying on a conversation or writing an email, you are consciously making decisions. However, your habits, drives, and instincts are all the province of the Middle Mind. These habits and drives develop quite differently from the conscious activities, and changing them is often quite difficult.

Consider our anatomy as an example of how the Middle Mind works. The portion of the brain that controls muscular activity such as balance and coordination is in the cerebellum.

When everything is operating correctly, we do not need to think to balance ourselves or coordinate our motor functions. The medulla oblongata controls the functions of the heart and the lungs, but we do not need to think, "I need to breathe in now" or "I need to breathe out now." Our body regulates these involuntary bodily responses.

Similarly, our everyday habits and drives are controlled by the Middle Mind in such a way that we are unaware of them. Problems arise, however, when the Middle Mind makes us act or feel in ways that are unhealthy or unwanted. The problem is exacerbated by the fact that in a battle between the Middle Mind and the conscious mind, the Middle Mind invariably wins. Thus, our bad habits or drives are difficult to overcome, even with the best of efforts. Step one in changing ourselves, our habits, and our drives means finding our way in to the Middle Mind. The vehicle to get there is hypnosis.

CHAPTER 8

HYPNOSIS AND HYPNOTHERAPY: MEANINGFUL DIFFERENCE

T wo key terms should be defined before we move forward. We have already used these terms extensively, but we need to make clear some important distinctions. The term *hypnosis* does not refer to a particular goal in and of itself when we discuss behavioral change. Being hypnotized is nothing more than a brief period of relaxation, unless there is some particular goal that is addressed during the act of hypnosis. Being placed under hypnosis will not overcome fear, nor will it stop a smoker from smoking. Hypnosis is a condition or state of your Middle Mind that is achieved through deep relaxation, producing a strong, narrow focus of attention combined with increased suggestibility. It is a deep relaxation, with various levels or depths. On the path we described in the previous chapter, it lives between sleep and the alert state of wakefulness, but it is distinct from both. A person in the deep state of relaxation is said to be "in a trance." The significance of a trance is measured in levels. By one measure, there are six levels of depth, and responsiveness to hypnotic suggestions and other conditions vary within each level.

We all have seen enough portrayals of Hollywood's fictional hypnosis to see the role that hypnosis can play in relaxation. What is new, however, to one who is first exposed to hypnosis is the narrow focus of the procedure. A hypnotized subject is fully cognizant of what the hypnotist is saying. He can hear and understand the words. He can respond to questions and other stimuli around him. He is not asleep, but he is very relaxed.

The key characteristic to hypnosis, however, is suggestibility. It is this suggestibility that serves as a tool to address long-held habits and drives at their very core. Once here, a person can receive suggestions and change behaviors.

So, if hypnosis is this narrowly-focused, suggestible point of relaxation, how can a hypnotic state be achieved? How do we narrow that focus and make proper suggestions upon which to change behavior? It is through hypnotherapy that we answer these questions.

Hypnotherapy is a therapeutic endeavor using hypnosis in which a therapist and a subject create a plan to address a problem. A person seeks a hypnotherapist because he has a problem. The therapist cannot help this person without a thorough understanding of that problem, examining its causes and effects upon the subject. With the therapist's help, the client outlines the goals he wants to reach, and the therapist then uses that information to design "suggestions" for hypnosis.

The real beauty of hypnotherapy is the speed with which success can be achieved in solving a client's problem. Hypnotherapy allows the client to deal immediately with the problem at the specific place where the problem is stored. Using all of our self-willed acts, our self-coaching, or our other talk therapies are like our efforts to fix the engine of a car without ever opening the hood. It is only guess-work, most of the time. A hypnotherapist knows how "to open the hood." The hood latch is popped with hypnotherapy. Once the engine, or our Middle Mind, is accessible, the right mechanic, or hypnotherapist, can guide a person to fix an array of engine (Middle Mind) issues. The wide range of access to the Middle Mind is why such an array of problems we describe in Part III can be addressed and solved, often very quickly.

The bottom line is to remember that hypnosis is a tool. A hypnotherapist is one who uses hypnosis as a tool to fine tune the Middle Mind. Hypnosis may be only a tool, but it is the key tool. The whole process of using this tool and the therapist's other skills and resources to achieve a client's goals is hypnotherapy.

CHAPTER 9

A BRIEF HISTORY
OF HYPNOSIS

Within the history of hypnosis there exists two misconceptions, both mingled with some truth. One misunderstanding is that it is an ancient activity with occult, religious, and mystical beginnings. The other is that hypnosis is a later development in history, involving new age, hippie-type origins. As Clark Hull put it in his book *Hypnosis and Suggestibility*, "All sciences alike have descended from magic and suggestions, but none has been so slow as hypnosis in shaking off the evil associations of its origins."

My theory as to how such misconceptions in the history of hypnosis developed is rather simple. The history of most medical treatments began with a single source: Louis Pasteur's work led to treatment for small pox; Jonas Salk developed the polio vaccine. In these cases, the development and treatment of these diseases can be traced back to a single person/persons. Throughout history, however, what we now call hypnosis came from diverse civilizations all over the planet, at various times and in different ways.

Each culture had those who observed and reflected on the phenomenon of what we term the *unconscious,* or what I am calling the Middle Mind. The science of hypnotherapy developed as these different people from far different cultures and different times worked to analyze the operations of the Middle Mind and to determine how to manipulate it. Of course, people did not consider hypnotherapy a science at the beginning. The religious were the earliest to claim it, and thus is became a spiritual tool for priests and temple leaders. Magicians thought they had discovered real magic. Greedy profiteers saw this developing tool as a real money maker, and hijacked it (or the illusion of it) for a money-making scheme. It was those with a more medical inclination who began to examine this idea of hypnosis as a type of therapy.

The roots of hypnosis are ancient. Cultures as old and distant as those of Sumatra, Persia, China, India, Egypt, Greece, and Rome used hypnosis in some form. Some Egyptian writings dating back to 1550 BC describe healing that used some form of hypnotic trance such as eye fixations. Other historians describe Indian Hindu "temple sleep" and Egyptian and Greek "sleep temples" as evidence of hypnosis which were religious tools for healing. These practices point to nascent hypnotic practices.

Confusion regarding hypnosis may well have started with the combination of two factors: the failure to recognize the existence and nature of Middle Mind and the misunderstanding of the "operator" of the cure or change in the hypnotic subject. Some contend the cause of a subject's change came from the stars or planets. Some "healers" argued that magnets were the tools needed to "heal" subjects who had problems. Others pointed to gods and spirits as the source of healing. The more brazen claimed that they themselves had the gifts or magic necessary to cure what ails people. It took millennia for scientists to realize that the main actor is the subject's own Middle Mind causing the change! Who knew? Apparently no one for the longest time.

It was not until the 1800s that studies began to grow around the idea of an individual's mind generating and creating change within itself. European physicians and early proponents of psychology began to hypothesize and test different theories concerning the consciousness and unconsciousness of people. Once they identified not only the mind as the location of the internal programming, but also that each individual served as the chief operator of his/her own mind, they then determined that it is the power of suggestion that works to effect the change. As they became more aware of the incredible ability of the Middle Mind, physicians began to use hypnosis to meet the needs of their patients. As early as the 1840s, surgeons were using hypnosis as anesthesia during major surgical operations. During the Civil War, hypnosis was widely used during amputations. With the advent of chemical anesthesia, however, hypnosis again fell into disuse.

Scottish ophthalmologist James Braid is considered the father of modern hypnosis. He coined the word *hypnosis* to distinguish it from mesmerism, magnetism, or hysteria, terms which had been attached to the less-than-scientific art of hypnotism. Braid would later regret using the term hypnosis because it connoted sleep, rather than the actual trance that occurs. His attempt to replace the term with *monoideism* (or single thought), however, came too late and did not take root.

Braid's attempt to change the term to *monoideism* actually denoted a most significant advancement of the science of hypnosis, as he was the first to state that hypnosis was psychological, disconnecting it from a treatment involving outside forces like magnets, spiritualists, and magicians. Braid was the first practitioner of psychosomatic medicine, in which a subject could be healed by his mind rather than the chemical.

Hypnosis advanced quickly in America during the twentieth century. Interest grew with the use of hypnosis to treat soldiers who suffered psychologically following the world wars and the Korean conflict. Today, we know that post-traumatic stress syndrome can affect more people than soldiers, and hypnosis has become an integral part of therapy.

As the interest in hypnosis grew, so did the general field of psychological studies. Hypnosis became an important field of research, and schools like Yale and Stanford led the way. Their work, in conjunction with the developments brought about by private practitioners in the healing sciences, helped define the terms of use and advance hypnosis as a legitimate field of practice and science. Even as the public may remain to some degree skeptical of hypnosis, science and the healing arts have embraced the practice, giving it a large stamp of approval.

Hypnosis continued to gain ground in the medical profession. In 1955, the British Medical Association approved hypnosis for treatment of neuroses and for use in surgery and childbirth, endorsing training in hypnosis for medical students and physicians. Three years later, the American Medical Association followed suit, as did the Canadian Medical

Association. In 1958, the Canadian Psychological Association endorsed hypnosis, followed by the American Psychological Association two years later. In 1961, the American Psychiatric Association added its endorsement, as well, to the practice of hypnosis.

From divergent and often bizarre beginnings, the journey to discovering the Middle Mind, how it works, and more importantly, how it can work to improve lives has reached a respected position, at least among professionals. Not just a parlor room trick any more, hypnosis is a legitimate practice, supported with over sixty years of endorsements.

CHAPTER 10

ENTERING THE MIDDLE MIND – MAKING SENSE OF HOW HYPNOSIS WORKS

The working of the mind is a complex process, not subject to a simple diagram with arrows and boxes. Where exactly in the brain the Middle Mind "operates" is still a mystery, for now. Experts have to reason backwards from effects to causes, and those causes, at least in the case of hypnosis, have taken a few thousand years to define. However, today we do know enough to access the Middle Mind and to work with it to effect change.

In order to explain the Middle Mind and show how hypnosis uses it to alter behavior, I will use the analogy of a computer, a machine with which most of us are familiar. While analogies can be useful in explaining the general ideas, bear in mind that all analogies will invariably break down at some point. For our purposes, though, the computer will serve to help us understand how hypnosis works.

First, consider the computer's internal system. It has a hard drive upon which all long term data is stored, even programs that are not in current use. A computer also requires Random Access Memory (RAM) in order to operate, a type of short term memory that allows quick access for immediate tasks. The RAM pulls up data from the hard drive for us in order to help us complete our tasks. The RAM then stores that information to the hard drive as each task is completed so that it can be retrieved later; it is a hardwired connection to your system.

Our subconscious, or Middle Mind, is our hard drive. The Middle Mind stores all data, our every memory since birth over the years. All of our years of education, our books, our loves, our hates are filed away in those layered memories. For me, years of near-meaningless baseball stats that I absorbed as a kid growing up are stored in my Middle Mind, as well as most of the dialogue to every episode of *Seinfeld*.

Our conscious mind, alert and active, is our RAM. It handles our immediate tasks at hand: our cooking, our reading, our driving needs.

Many programs essential to the computer's operation are engaged and working without a user's knowledge. These programs are equivalent to the Middle Mind's operations. Our drives, habits, and instincts work along the same principle; they work without our conscious awareness of them.

However, our analogy of the computer breaks down as soon as we discuss the need for repair. If a computer program or its data becomes corrupted, we can take steps to uninstall the corrupted program and replace it with a healthy one. Behavior problems in the Middle Mind, however, require a different approach. Our Middle Mind programs that lead to poor diet decisions, or create a fear of even the friendliest dog, or make sleep difficult cannot simply be uninstalled with the click of a computer key. Like many of today's toughest computer viruses, the fix may not be simple. Until the advancement of recent "decoders" in hypnotherapy, people might have a life sentence of frustrating behaviors, or at best, lifetimes of constant battles with themselves resulting in yo-yo diets, on-again-off-again smoking, or medicating before flying. Some have sought help in long-term traditional psychological therapy treatments. Hypnosis, however, is the modern key to help and to change.

Let's try another analogy. When we drive a car, we think of ourselves as making all the decisions. Actually, much of the operation of a car – the work of the engine, the safety features, the climate controls, the warning alarms – are all active and essential to the proper functioning of a modern vehicle. If the car breaks down, our sitting in the driver's seat and simply willing the car to be fixed will not achieve anything (although I am sure most of us have tried "reasoning" with a car at some point). The first big step in getting the car operational is to look under the hood. Think of hypnosis as the latch to opening the hood to our Middle Minds. Once inside, we can begin to take steps to correct the problem.

CHAPTER 11

CHANGING THE MIDDLE MIND FOR GOOD

The key benefit of hypnotherapy, other than it simply works, is that its results come quickly and the results are permanent. Let us now look generally at the steps in successful hypnotherapy. Each person is different and each challenge facing that person is different, so we can offer only a broad framework of what to expect during hypnotherapy. If you are new to hypnotherapy, here is what you can expect.

The first goal of the hypnotherapist is to know his client. The therapist will be interested in your age, family life, educational background, work history, likes and dislikes, and personal interests. Eventually, the therapist will focus his attention on the conditions for which help is sought. You and your therapist will talk about the nature of the problem and the desired outcomes you are looking for. The therapist will want to know your history of the problem, your battles with it, and your prior attempts to overcome it. You may discuss the causes of the problem, but there is a strong distinction between hypnotherapy and other approaches, such as psychotherapy. Many other behavioral therapists focus on the origins of a problem with the intention of unearthing past triggering events in order to heal the here and now. Hypnotherapy, however, provides a very confident, future-oriented approach. The hypnotherapist may not dismiss or ignore a past event. In fact, in some cases the therapist may offer specific strategies for dealing with the residue of original causes or events. Hypnotherapy, however, is a tool that can change the future without dwelling on or in the past. It is a unique approach in its future orientation.

Another focus of the hypnotherapist in the first meeting is the observation of the way the client communicates, both verbally and nonverbally. The goal will be to speak the client's language. If the overall goal is to change that "little voice" in your head, it needs to be phrased so that you readily understand the new voice.

From these early observations the hypnotherapist will work with you in developing a game plan to achieve your goals. The game plan, among other things, will possibly address developing aversions to behavior/thinking associated with the problematic behavior and in creating positive responses to improved behavior. In my case, these aversions centered on foods I needed to avoid instinctively. I also needed a whole new mindset when faced with vegetables and other beneficial foods, and I needed to lower my caloric intake and to be happy doing so. This game plan then becomes the suggestions which will be essential in the ongoing hypnotherapy process.

After the initial session, client and therapist will use later sessions to discuss progress, the focus of the problem, and any new thoughts or experiences a client may have that may be relevant to the game plan. Session by session, your therapy will mature or refine as your Middle Mind gets fine-tuned. Usually, a session will end with a brief use of hypnosis of no more than ten to fifteen minutes. Because the therapist will use relaxation to introduce the hypnosis, he will adjust the setting, muting external sounds and light, and possibly adding light background music. Throughout the sessions, the therapist will speak quietly, peacefully, and slowly. The loud, boisterous, demanding voices often characterizing Hollywood's depiction of hypnotism or the outlandish showmanship of stage hypnotists have no place in real client-oriented, objective-focused hypnotherapy. A client is involved from the first step in changing his game plan, and he will remain in control throughout the entire process.

Having never been hypnotized before, I wondered if I were even been under any hypnosis as I began my sessions. I still heard and understood every word my therapist was saying. I was aware of everything that was happening, and I was in full control of all of my faculties and my decision-making. Never did I become unconscious, like sleep or chemical anesthesia produces, which I now realize is a state of mind very different from that of the Middle Mind. In time, I realized two things: First, during sessions, I was highly focused on both the issue I was dealing with and the voice of my therapist. As James Braid's term *monoideism* suggests, the process creates a highly relaxed state that permits a single (mono) thought (idea) to be the sole focus for the hypnotized subject. Second, the changes that hypnosis worked in me were subtle, yet profound. I began to make better decisions about my eating. I avoided those foods which were unhealthy for me, and I enjoyed foods that were better for me. Attempting new vegetables became almost an obsession, and I loved the new tastes I was experiencing. I paid closer attention to my food intake, and my entire approach to eating became more balanced and sensible. I began to view food as a fuel source and my body as an engine that I wanted to keep running smoothly, as it was manufactured to do.

As so often happens, one action impacting my behavior created unanticipated rewards. One simple reward, but a profound one in my case, is that as my diet became cleaner, my palate became cleaner, as well. My ability to taste and enjoy the natural and healthy foods improved dramatically. An apple or a tangerine made my taste buds dance, rather than the chips and dips to which I had grown accustomed. Bananas rather than chocolate have now become nature's candy to me. But it was not only the enjoyment of the food that changed. My clothes fit so much better. I felt so much better. I could move more freely because my joints functioned like those of a teenager! My confidence soared with all of these changes.

During a therapy session, once you are relaxed and focused, the hypnotherapist will provide you with suggestions culled from your earlier discussions. The Middle Mind does not work logically; with suggestions, we are simply adding new ingredients to the recipe. The Middle Mind, in its own extraordinary way will take these suggestions (ingredients) and use them to create new behaviors. Hypnotherapists themselves marvel at the Middle Mind's incredible ability to alter our behaviors so quickly and efficiently.

Clients experience different depths or levels of hypnosis. Hypnotherapists can monitor your depth level by observing you and your responses. The ability to enter into a hypnotic trance quickly and the ability to reach deeper depths of hypnosis vary from person to person. The good news is that for many behavioral changes, the slightest levels of hypnosis are sufficient to effect changes. I assume, in looking back on my first experiences as a subject, that I was in a light trance. I really did not believe that I had been hypnotized, rather that I was just agreeably cooperating with Ken. In retrospect, I am sure that my level of relaxation combined with my singular focus on his voice and my cooperation with his suggestions all indicate that I in fact had been hypnotized. In later sessions, I experienced even deeper relaxation and characteristics of deeper levels of hypnosis. With each succeeding session, two things will happen. First, a client relaxes faster, leading to a speedier entrance into a hypnotic state. Second, a client experiences a deeper level of hypnosis. As a result, clients make quicker progress with each session.

Sessions are just the first step to successful changes in behavior. The therapist may record the hypnosis portion of a session and then instruct the client on how to use the recordings to achieve behavioral changes. The goal is not to simply change. The goal is to make a permanent change. Think of it as creating "muscle memory" for the Middle Mind. Every repetition is reinforcement. Every repetition builds permanence. No client wants to go through this effort for a temporary change. For me, my yo-yo dieting was over!

Besides the follow-up sessions with the recordings, clients must apply their newfound behavioral changes regularly. For the dieter, these changes mean dealing with the daily food intake and monitoring the correct foods in the correct amounts. For a smoker who is trying to quit, changes mean addressing those cues that trigger the desire for a cigarette. For someone dealing with an irrational fear of heights, the changes mean facing the tests of elevators, escalators, or other challenges that the therapist outlines.

All of these applications secure the changes that a client desires. They also, session by session, measure the progress a client is making. The therapist will help pinpoint weekly progress, record the history, and help to refine or tailor each session and the post-therapy session applications. With each session, the client will begin to see changes happen. As behavior changes, confidence grows. Soon, the client will boldly embrace the new behaviors and rejoice at each new benchmark he reaches.

CHAPTER 12

HYPNOTHERAPY MISCELLANY: LIMITATIONS, MOTIVATIONS, CHANGE

As excited as I get about the broad applications of this practice and its amazing results that I have witnessed, hypnotherapy is not a magic cure-all for every human ill or challenge. It is not a simple "snap your fingers and you're all better now" approach to whatever ails mankind. In these next sections, we will look at some of the basic misconceptions and limitations of this practice.

Hypnotherapy does not offer a cure for mental illness. It cannot end schizophrenia, bipolar disorder, or personality disorders. Some symptoms of depression can be alleviated with hypnotherapy, but because serious clinical depression may have a chemical or organic cause or may indicate a more serious mental illness, therapists proceed cautiously. If you suffer with depression, certainly consult with a hypnotherapist about your symptoms, however.

One of the early problems with the use of hypnosis as therapy resulted from its use with mental illness. When hypnosis failed to work, its effectiveness was questioned. Only when researchers determined that the most appropriate candidates for hypnotherapy were sane, stable persons of reasonable intelligence that the amazing breadth of hypnotherapy began to be truly understood.

Others with whom hypnosis is not particularly effective include people of extremely low intelligence. Their lack of cognizance makes understanding and following suggestions difficult. Since the foundation of hypnosis is communication, those challenged in hearing and comprehending language are at an extreme disadvantage, as well.

Besides communication, another key trait for a person undergoing hypnotherapy is the ability to trust. A client's initial step in undergoing hypnosis is to relax, and in order to relax, he must trust the therapist. People with paranoia or people who have trouble trusting even trustworthy people are not good candidates for hypnosis-based therapy.

Some of the best candidates for hypnotherapy are those who have experienced coaching in one form or another, such as in athletics, drama, music, or in organizations such as the Boy Scouts or Girl Scouts. The success of hypnotherapy requires motivation and commitment. People who have already made such commitments through coaching understand the concept of suggestions and behavioral change.

As much as I would love to be in a position to simply give away the benefits of hypnosis (I am not, by the way), free hypnotherapy would likely fail. As I heard Dr. Crow once say, the client needs to have "skin in the game." Payment for service reinforces a client's sense of obligation and commitment to succeed. The higher the motivation for change at the beginning translates into greater success throughout the whole process for the client, much like the goal of winning does for those who have undergone coaching. Making a large payment to undergo therapy was a large motivation for me to follow through, and, in retrospect, the success I experienced helped make my cost a real bargain!

Motivation needs to be matched with a certain level of discipline. Success in hypnotherapy is not achieved and measured within a session. It is within real life where the change is tested and experienced daily. Principles addressed in sessions need to be applied regularly. Throughout the process, a therapist will assign "homework," or steps to follow to achieve the goals that are set during the sessions. These steps are necessary to success and permanency of the change.

Counter-motivations may hinder some people in their progress and in the worst case may actually sabotage the entire process. Sometimes the therapist will recognize this resistance during the hypnotherapy and can deal with it. At other times, a client may cling to the resistance too tightly, destroying efforts to change. Remember, a therapist never controls the client. The client cannot be made to do anything he does not want to do. A man seeking to lose weight who simply refuses to drop his two beers a night (and the calories that go with them) is destined to fail because his unreasonable stubbornness controls the entire process.

This control that a client exercises, on the other hand, should comfort a person considering hypnotherapy. One can trust the therapist to an even greater degree if the therapist is no threat.

As we will see in the chapter ahead, a hypnotherapist cannot make a person do anything against his will. No one can be led to act contrary to his existing morals or nature. A hypnotherapist lacks authority to make a saint into a sinner or a sinner into a saint.

When a client makes changes to his behavior, how "locked in" or permanent are those changes? Will a client regress in his progress?

Since the client has learned this problematic behavior over time, there is always a future risk that the client may experience of some type of re-emergence of that behavior. Some changes are more permanent than others. Some behavioral changes are as near to permanent as they can be, but others, not so much. Let me illustrate the differences.

One behavior I had to address and change was my aversion to foods that are good for me, such as foods lower in calories, particularly vegetables. I accomplished that goal, and rather quickly too, I might add. Before my attitude change, even the appearance of broccoli coming near my plate filled me with revulsion. Afterwards, I eagerly anticipated broccoli, as well as other vegetables. Those changes are clearly permanent and unchangeable. I cannot imagine not enjoying these tasty, low-calorie foods the rest of my life.

The change in my behavior that led to my love of broccoli was a new adventure in my behavior and diet. I developed an active desire to try new, healthy foods. These new tastes rewarded my attempts and reinforced my experimentation with healthy nutrition. Like my newfound love for broccoli, I do not see myself losing this new behavior of experiencing new "eats."

The greatest challenge proved to be creating aversions to unhealthy and high calorie foods. Since childhood, I have formed desires for burgers, fried chicken, sweets of all kinds, and pizza. Pre-hypnotherapy, I consumed far too many diet sodas (that actually inhibit weight loss and are full of ingredients hazardous to our health). I have systematically dealt with these behaviors during my therapy, and I have made significant changes. However, all of those years of consuming those unhealthy foods still fill my memory banks, and they always will. They will never completely disappear, I suppose. In many cases, those memories are tied to pleasant events. Repeating similar events may tend to trigger occasions for relapses. I continue with a wariness about consuming those unhealthy foods. The positive news is that the aversions that I created do prevail and the challenges never appear too great. I am confident of life-long success in these behavioral changes, as well.

One final point that needs to be highlighted is that many changes may occur other than just behaviors. I remember hearing an interview with the late, great Pat Sumerall. Pat was the voice of the National Football League on CBS for years. He also covered the Masters Invitational Golf Tournaments, as well as other great sporting events after his years with the NFL. He also drank too much, ultimately entering rehabilitation for his alcoholism. Blessedly, he had success in overcoming his addiction, or at least in controlling it. In his interview, he addressed the changes he had to make in his lifestyle. He said the one thing that he learned is that he had to change his playground and his playmates. He could no longer frequent some places (bars) and hang out with his drinking buddies.

As part of the hypnotherapy success, you may experience changes two ways. One change may be the new practices adopted as part of the active consultation with your therapist. The other changes may occur as more of a side effect of the positive changes brought about by the hypnotherapy. In either case, you should not resist these changes, but embrace them. If your ultimate goal is sound and your motivations right, your success will be filled with many positives changes

CHAPTER 13

MYTHS AND MISCONCEPTIONS

The general population and pop culture as a whole hold a considerable number of myths and misconceptions about hypnosis and hypnotherapy. The ancient and diverse lineage of the use of mind "therapy," though used as a wonderful treatment tool, is so full of wonder and mystery that it has become a popular topic for media reporting and fictional works. In more modern times, it has become a topic fit for screen, stage, and of course, caricature. As a result, the public has some fairly universal misconceptions about hypnosis which impact the general view of hypnotherapy. Starting with a fairly exhaustive list of these myths and misunderstandings culled from Robin Butterfield's *Hidden Depths: The Story of Hypnosis*, let us address the most common misconceptions.

1. You are asleep when you are hypnotized. Historically, a hypnotic trance has been associated with "non-consciousness" and the only conclusion was that it must be some form of sleep. Because we have different degrees of alertness, it was assumed that sleep also had different degrees; many considered the hypnotic stage as just one of them. As we pointed out in our earlier descriptions of the Middle Mind, the better description for the place of hypnosis is in a separate non-sleep, non-conscious mind, a third category all on its own.

Consciousness is characterized by an alertness to the tasks at hand and an awareness of various competing stimuli. Sleep is characterized by relaxation without an awareness of surroundings. The hypnotic trance generally requires deep relaxation, thus its similarity to sleep. But there is a sharp awareness and focus on one particular thought to the exclusion of all other sensory activity in hypnosis that is lacking in sleep. Therefore, it is not sleep. The hypnotized subject is well aware of what is going on around him. (There is a form of hypnotic trance in which the subject is not in a relaxed state, but we will save that for another chapter.)

This idea of hypnosis as sleep may be what leads to a similar misconception, that to be hypnotized a person must keep his eyes closed and remain completely still. Actually, neither is required. Because relaxation is step one in the process, some people will simply close their eyes at the beginning of the process (I always did), or a therapist may request that a client do so. To me, it just made sense to help facilitate the process. If a subject begins the hypnotic transition with his eyes open, as he relaxes it is natural for him to close his eyes as he relaxes.

Nor should a subject worry about remaining absolutely still. The goal is comfort in order to accentuate relaxation. Just as we remain relatively still to fall asleep, it makes sense to reduce movement to help the hypnotic process. Mummification, however, is not necessary. And yes, you may scratch that itch without fear of reprisal!

2. You are unconscious under hypnosis. Unfortunately, I have had the occasion to be under chemical anesthesia a number of times in my life, starting with a tonsillectomy at six years old and including two wrist surgeries in high school, several eye procedures, and of course the biggie I discussed in the earlier chapters of this book. I am always amazed at how that time just disappears between my counting backwards from one hundred in the operating room and awaking in the recovery room. My preconceived notion was that hypnosis would be similar to that experience, or to sleep, or to some other weird state I have never experienced before. I won't say that I was disappointed that the Middle Mind turned out to be familiar ground, similar to my near-sleep or daydreams, but it was not a Disney-style fantasyland full of magic either. One thing is certain, however; I was not unconscious.

3. You are under the power of the hypnotherapist. This myth is a serious error that Hollywood has perpetuated through its films. Hollywood may not be without some basis for its error, however, since the earliest pioneers of hypnotherapy operated on similar misconceptions themselves. At the turn of the century society was more fragmented with castes, classes, and cultural mandates of submissiveness between masters and servants. This stratification influenced those seeking to master the art of hypnosis to assume a more authoritarian role as therapist. Their view was that while in a hypnotic state, the patient could be ordered to change his or her behavior and that the Middle Mind would follow the directive. In different societies and cultures, such a view may have had some effect, but it was not the key element that creates the success of today's hypnotherapy.

In the early twentieth century, American psychiatrist Milton Erickson, the father of modern hypnotherapy, pioneered the permissive hypnosis style of treatment. Erickson grasped the concept that the Middle Mind does not respond the way the conscious mind does to directions. The Middle Mind takes suggestions and uses those suggestions to develop changed behavior. The Middle Mind will not be told what it must do.

As a result, we now know the hypnotherapist is not exerting power upon a client; rather he is working cooperatively with the client on his plans and goals for change. The hypnotherapist shows great respect for the client and seeks to exude gentleness. The clients' beliefs and language are paramount in developing the individual approach to therapy. The goal is to empower the client's Middle Mind to find its own solution to the problem.

A related misconception is that the hypnotists dominate gullible people. We now realize that successful behavior change only occurs with intellectual and intelligible cooperation between the therapist and the subject. The idea of dominance or gullibility, thus, loses all logical support. Actually, the sharper and more cooperative the client, the faster the progress toward the goal.

4. Hypnosis is dangerous. Hypnosis would be useless as a tool of treatment if it did not work. Even knowledgeable detractors agree that the evidence overwhelmingly supports the science and efficacy of hypnosis as a tool of behavioral change.

Hypnosis actually enhances the speed with which behavior is modified and improved, but as with any therapy, whether physical or psychological, precautions are always advised. Take for example the open heart procedure I described in CHAPTER 2. I permitted the physicians to anesthetize me, to open my chest, and to detach my heart from my body. A man actually reached into my chest and held my heart. I trusted all kinds of pharmaceutical manufacturers, doctors, and nurses to keep me alive. Surrounded with potential risks while I was totally unconscious, I acted on trust and faith in the true professionals.

Although hypnosis can be used in both useful and useless ways, it comes with far fewer risks than typical health treatments. Why? Because a patient is in control the entire time and has the ability to exit a trance whenever she wants.

Think of hypnotherapy as electricity or fire. Under control, these are most trustworthy tools for generating heat, cooking food, or clearing underbrush. Qualified hypnotherapists ensure that their clients are well treated and emotionally cared for with dignity and respect. The same steps you take to protect yourself when employing other professionals, whether in health care, financial care, or dry cleaning, you should take with hypnotherapists. Are the ones you are considering both qualified and trustworthy? If you can answer those questions with confidence, you are set to begin.

As with any area in life, unscrupulous characters can, too, be expected to exist in the hypnotherapy field. If in doubt, don't go. Get to know your hypnotherapist, and make sure that you trust him or her. And avoid those stage hypnotists! They are our next subject.

5. Hypnosis makes you cluck like a chicken: the sorry case of stage hypnotists. I must admit, most of what I thought about hypnotism came from watching snippets of stage hypnotists on television. I had never seen one in person, and I really do not remember spending much time in viewing their performances on TV, but I had obviously seen enough to have formed some hard and fast (and very wrong) ideas about hypnosis. I never believed professional wrestling was real, and I never trusted that TV faith healers were truly healing anyone. Looking back, I was the fool to have thought of stage hypnotism as much more than showmanship and audience manipulation.

This is not to say that stage hypnotists are incapable of performing hypnosis, but it is highly unlikely, given the setting and the time constraints of an entertainment program. A full hypnotic induction typically takes time and patience. Since the primary first step is relaxation, a performance setting does not present the best accommodations for hypnosis.

So, how do they do it? At a theater or a club, the performer may employ a short-cut technique of pressing the carotid artery just behind the ear to produce something that looks like a trance; it is, however, just dizziness. More likely, he has planted several people in the audience known as "horses" in the industry. These may simply be actors. It is possible that the horses are associates of the performer whom he knows to be really good subjects for hypnosis and whom he has hypnotized repeatedly before. These horses will jump to the front of the line when the hypnotist asks for volunteers from the audience. Among the volunteers, the stage hypnotist will, with some simple test, determine which are highly suggestible, meaning not necessarily that they will be hypnotized, but rather that they follow and imitate the actions of the horses. These followers are ones who are happy to go on stage and be part of the fun. Think choreographed peer pressure. Sadly, some entertainers will just make participants look silly, and still others demean the whole experience with lewd acts.

Remember two key points that we know are true about real hypnosis. First, a person is not unconscious and is always aware of what is going on. Secondly, the subject of the hypnotic trance still remains in control of his actions.

Stories abound of charlatan stage performers. In his autobiography, Mark Twain tells of being a volunteer to such a performer and how that performer handled Twain's challenges. Another author writes about a community leader who played along only to deck the hypnotist upon being awakened because he knew exactly what the performer had done, and he was embarrassed by his own actions.

These performers use the mystique of hypnosis as a guise for their scams. Remember, their goals are entertainment, particularly laughter, accolades, and promotion for their shows. Any embarrassment or harm that may result from his show is of little concern to them.

A strict code of ethics guides true hypnotherapists. Their sole objective is helping their clients safely, confidently, and privately achieve behavioral changes that positively affect their daily lives.

6. Hypnosis is a magical power. Because the effects of hypnosis and early hypnotherapy were observed without people understanding the means by which change was wrought, hypnosis could certainly have appeared to those early observers to be magical, spiritual, or ethereal. It was difficult to explain, both by hypnotists and their subjects alike.

As a result, the purveyors of the arts and sciences were left to claim all sorts of causes for the cure. Those who sought to use it for entertainment, accolades, power, or profits were capable of claiming special magical gifts, and they were left alone to do so. Different religious operators assigned the power to their gods, operating through their institution and their priorities.

Today, we better grasp the workings of hypnosis as a tool of change, and we realize that it is not magic at all. Admittedly, the science still fascinates us, and we know that we have much more to learn about how the mind converts suggestions under hypnosis into remarkably changed behavior, but we grasp enough of how this marvelous tool works to make practical use of it.

As a successful subject of hypnotherapy, I must admit that in describing my changed behavior to others, I would say, "It's magical!" My choice of phrase was based on two reasons. My view of hypnotherapy was nothing like I thought it would be. I was always alert, never unconscious. I was always in control of my senses. At first, I actually thought that nothing was really happening to me. But, then, the weirdest things began to happen. I describe them as subtle changes, but really my altered behavior was quite remarkable. My desire to eat healthy foods, particularly vegetables, was a completely new experience. My ability to avoid the high calorie, low nutrition diet of my past was evidence of a self-control that I had not had before. And my overall commitment to the weight loss program and the reorientation of my entire behavior was just . . . well, what can I say, but seemingly magical.

Now that I know more of the science of hypnotherapy, I get it. However, I still remain in complete awe of its usefulness to change behaviors and change lives.

7. Hypnosis alone is therapy. While I have addressed this misconception earlier in more detail (CHAPTER 8), this discussion will offer a quick summary. Hypnosis is remarkable, but it is only a tool. A subject gains nothing substantial other than maybe a period of rejuvenation or relaxation from being hypnotized, similar to a good nap. Hypnosis become therapeutic and capable of facilitating change only in combination with other elements. The therapist and the client must establish a strong relationship built on trust and fostered in a comfortable atmosphere. Together, the pair must examine the history of the problem behavior and then reach an agreement on the targeted goals. The therapist must take the objectives of the agreement and develop a script of suggestions to use during the sessions. Then the therapist must guide the client from relaxation into hypnosis and into an adequate level of trance depth. In the language of the client and with highly structured signals, the therapist must offer the appropriate suggestions and encouragements which the client's Middle Mind will digest and utilize to reprogram behavior. In all likelihood, the therapist will phrase the words so that the client may reinforce the changes at home following the session. The therapist will then correctly bring the client out of hypnosis in such a way that the gains which the client has made will be optimized.

Hypnosis is key to success in hypnotherapy. But only in the hands of a trained hypnotherapist can hypnosis accelerate the permanent behavior change.

8. Some people cannot be hypnotized. This statement may actually have some truth in it. But while some people do not make good candidates for hypnosis, most do.

Some persons are mentally incapable of being hypnotized. Since hypnotism is based on language communication, anything that interferes with that communication limits hypnotism's effectiveness. Many mental disorders restrict hypnosis. Those who suffer serious paranoia are not good candidates since hypnotism requires a high level of trust in the therapist. Persons with very low IQs are less likely to have success with hypnotism, also, since their ability to reason through to change is diminished.

So, what about the extremely bright subject? Are they too intelligent to fall under hypnosis? Will not their power of rationalization overwhelm the hypnotic process? Actually, the more bright and creative a person is, the more likely he or she is to be a good candidate for hypnosis and successful hypnotherapy. Highly motivated people also make strong candidates.

Even the lightest depths of hypnosis can foster successful hypnotherapy, and just about any mentally balanced person can reach these levels.

Since true hypnosis places the subject in charge of his behavior, no one can be hypnotized if he does not want to be.

In very rare cases, serious fears or misconceptions about the process can actually block hypnosis. In such cases, some pre-hypnosis exploration and education may be of great value in the process.

9. People may get stuck in a trance for a long time, maybe permanently. Remember, in hypnosis, the subject remains in control of himself and can exit the trance at any time. In fact, hypnotic trances are very similar to the trances we are in as we daydream, drive somewhere without thinking about the drive, or get lost in a book. Just as we can exit any of these common trances, we can exit an hypnotic trance. And we do not have to consciously act to exit a trance. Just as a night's sleep will come to an end with a natural awakening at some point without an alarm, a person will naturally leave the pleasant hypnotic oasis of the Middle Mind.

10. Emergencies could occur during hypnosis, or my therapist departs leaving the trance in place. These misconceptions are somewhat related. The first deals with the concern of an emergency occurring during a client's hypnotic state, a therapist having a heart attack or some other health crisis, for example, that leaves him unable to function. At the risk of sounding repetitious, I say again that people under hypnosis are always in control. Clients control their journeys to their Middle Minds. Every person is very aware of the conditions he may find himself in, just as if an emergency occurred on the drive along the expressway while his mind was lost in thought. Just as a person's mind can shift gears instantly to protect him, it can also shift focus during hypnosis.

Let me share a somewhat embarrassing story that happened to me during a hypnotherapy session for my weight loss to illustrate the point. I had scheduled a 2:30 p.m. appointment. That morning I had two lengthy meetings. I ate lunch and washed it down with a bit more water than usual, too much water actually just preceding a session. I'm sure you can see where this is going. Upon my arrival, I weighed in. We had our typical discussion of the past week in which we evaluated how I was progressing in my dieting and behaviors, how I was handling any challenges that I faced, and what areas I could work on during hypnosis and in the week to come. Near the end of the hour, we began the induction. Of course, stage one is relaxation and a narrowing of focus. At this particular point, I had a sudden and immediate call of nature. I was already moving into a light trance, but I was cognizant enough of my bladder to pop out of the trance, somewhat to my therapist's surprise, and explain my situation. He understood completely. I excused myself briefly and took care of business. After returning, I completed my session. This story does have a happy ending. We decided to recheck my weight after my "water loss" and, sure enough, I had lost another half a pound!

A somewhat related misconception is that the only person who can bring a person out of a trance is the person who puts him into a trance. As my illustration highlights, no one needs assistance to exit a trance, and certainly in the event of an emergency situation, others could enter the picture and awaken you, if necessary.

11. People can be hypnotized from distances or even from video devices like TV. This misconception impacted me.

During my very skeptical period, I always avoided eye contact with the hypnotherapists I encountered regularly. Really! I just was not willing to take any chances. Why? I had seen the movie *Now You See Me* about a group of Robin Hood- type magicians who do "bad" for good. In that movie, Woody Harrelson plays a very talented hypnotist capable of entrancing a subject instantly, even from across a room. Of course, this Hollywood portrayal is completely false and impractical. True hypnosis takes patience, relaxation, and a hefty amount of trust from the client. Hypnosis from across a room or through a TV is impossible, no matter what stage or screen may portray.

12. Pocket watches and stares are tools of hypnosis. Pop culture has many believing that with an evil eye or snake eyes, a dominant doctor can use his gaze to bring a trance upon an unsuspecting victim. In many cases, the evil stare is used in conjunction with the pocket watch and an enjoinment to "Follow the watch." These techniques both raise somewhat similar concerns. A dominant stare certainly can make anyone uncomfortable and can create conscious concerns, but there is no concern of being hypnotized. We might have some other psychological reaction to such behavior, but it will not be a hypnotic trance.

The swinging watch actually does have some historical basis in hypnosis. As a technique to encourage relaxation, eye open fixation on a spot can help. Although it is not often used today, it is a technique still in use. Patients should not expect to run into this method, but it should not be of any concern either. Once again, a patient in hypnotherapy is always in control and is well aware of all things going on.

13. Hypnosis can cure any ailment. The possibilities of behavioral help with hypnotherapy abound, but cures for any and all ailments, mental or physical, are not limitless. Physical ailments of a real material physical or chemical origin cannot be cured by hypnotherapy. For illustration, I will use extreme analogies. A decapitated arm cannot be restored or even reattached with hypnotherapy. (Hypnotherapy can help deal with the "ghost pain" from a lost limb, but that will be discussed in CHAPTER 19.) A drunken person cannot escape the hangover that follows a binge until the chemicals clear the body.

However, where there exists a behavioral activity that leads to a physical ailment, hypnosis and therapy can change the underlying drives or habits. An ethical hypnotherapist will require that medical specialists have determined that the physical cause of an issue has been addressed before pursuing hypnotherapy.

With particular reference to pain, hypnotherapy can provide quite credible relief in situations where traditional medical treatment has not been successful. In fact, an early use of hypnosis that is now gaining new interest is the use of this incredible tool in the place of chemical anesthesia. Dr. Crow, my instructor, popularized the term "hypnothesia," and he has trained many physicians in the technique. Ken Thompson, my personal hypnotherapist, underwent cataract surgery and a colonoscopy using only hypnosis and forgoing chemical anesthesia.

We are learning with each passing day how individual attitudes, beliefs, and psychologies influence the development and course of any disease. Everyone generally understands that people with sunny dispositions seem to have healthier and happier lives. As researchers continue to understand the connection between the physical and mental, it is certainly likely that hypnotherapy will play an increasing role in the prevention and cure of sickness.

14. Hypnosis can cause dangerous after effects. Sessions with a reputable, well-trained, and ethical hypnotherapist make this concern nearly impossible. For explanation, let us turn to some computer analogies.

You may be familiar with the phrase, "Garbage In, Garbage Out" or GIGO. Like a computer, if we input only negative suggestions, then theoretically only the negative will result. So, if hypnosis is practiced carelessly or maliciously, as with some stage hypnosis acts seeking only entertainment and profit, then there may be some adverse after effects. It is conceivable that a hypnotists working with a self-destructive subject (one seeking and agreeing to enhance poor behavior) could achieve dangerous results. I have seen no evidence of such results, but theoretically it is possible.

Also, like a computer, hypnosis is best conducted in a systematic manner. When a computer powers down normally, it shuts down its programs in a specific order for a specific purpose. A sudden loss of power may require remedial steps in rebooting the computer. Most modern computers can handle these sudden interruptions, and people under hypnosis can, as well. But, to insure the well-being of the client, a hypnotherapist will want to systematically bring a client out of her trance. The therapist is achieving two things with a smooth transition. First, the therapist insures the well-being of her client. Second, the beneficial gains of the session are preserved and reinforced as the trance ends.

15. I can hypnotize myself for the same gains. Self-hypnosis and hypnotherapy with an experienced practitioner are quite different. I am a big fan of self-hypnosis, but one cannot expect the same gains and depth of the changes that come from working with a professional. The best order of practice is to experience hypnosis with a professional. Depth of trance and breadth of application are both better with a hypnotherapist. The accelerated changes in behavior only happen together.

Also, the exposure to hypnosis that is performed correctly will create a standard and expectation for a client as she considers self-hypnosis. A therapist may very well encourage self-hypnosis and instruct her client as to the proper methods of the process. Maybe most importantly, she may show her client how to reinforce the behavioral gains that have been made under her care.

16. Hypnosis is the same as meditation. While these two practice may appear similar, there are numerous differences. First, and most evident, is the fact that hypnosis involves two people. The act is a cooperative experience planned in advance. Meditation generally involves one person.

Second, the trance of hypnosis is a much different state of mind than the one in meditation. The meditative state is really just mind-cleared relaxation with no goal or instruction. Either the mind is empty of thought or the mind is left to wander. The trance of hypnotherapy begins with relaxation, and as one enters the Middle Mind, most conscious thoughts will be dispensed with, but not all. The hypnotic trance leaves the client focused on a specific line of thought, but it is not simply a random thought. It is a line of thought that the therapist and the client have agreed upon and have planned for. The hypnotherapist works in concert with the client to help her relax and focus on the target.

Testing of the brain during meditation and during hypnosis highlights the differences. In meditation, the brain becomes less active. In hypnosis, part of the brain actually increases its activity. This activity is located in the brain's frontal lobe, considered the seat of emotion in the brain. Such research into this connection helps to reinforce the idea that people cannot simply think themselves into new behavior.

Other than relaxation and the benefits derived from it, meditation is without objectives. Hypnotherapy, on the other hand, is very goal-directed and intentional.

17. Under hypnosis people can accurately recall things that happened earlier in their lives, even past lives. Our brains are incredible machines, and the capacity to retain data is vast. These amazing hard drives we have will accumulate and retain basically all of our life experiences. Recalling them, however, is often difficult. Hypnosis can be used to reach back into the data and fetch this old data. The relaxation allows entrance through the Middle Mind to the warehouse of the brain. Think of the focus achieved during hypnotherapy as the flashlight we might use to focus along the corridor of stored information. Hypnosis is an amazing tool to reach this data, and depending on the objectives of therapy, the recalling of memories may be of particular use.

However, these retrieved memories may not be fully accurate. Just as computer data may be corrupted, so, too, data in our memories may manifest falsehoods. This can happen several ways. The original recordings of these memories may be inaccurate themselves. Or something may have corrupted the memory while it was in storage. Or the memory may be altered in the process of retrieval. Besides our actual memory, the brain is storing our daydreams, fantasies, and other less-than-accurate ideas. Could these bleed into our actual memories?

Because of these potential issues with memories and hypnosis, courts of law do not allow memories reached during hypnosis to be used in court proceedings. Law enforcement, therefore, is reluctant to use hypnosis as what one might think is a great investigative tool for fear that all of a witness's testimony will be excluded in court.

With regard to past lives memory, all I can say is that such claims are bogus. Someone's claim to have traveled back to prior ages simply proves the limitations of past memory recall in hypnosis. Mind you, age regression and memory recall are effective tools when they are used reasonably in therapeutic settings where changed behavior is the objective, but such tools should be used only in light of their limitations.

18. People under hypnosis can be made to tell the truth (or lie). Let us assume for this discussion that we are talking about telling the truth or telling a lie under duress. We must return to our hypnosis fundamentals again to address this misconception. A person in a hypnotic trance is well aware of everything that is going on during the session. In fact, as to the sole idea or thought that the hypnosis is centered upon, the subject is actually hyper-focused. The subject is in control of his thinking and his will. The hypnotist at no point can override a person's will. Therefore, a person cannot be made to speak the truth if he does not want to speak the truth, or to lie if he does not want to lie.

19. Hypnosis can produce paranormal powers. Let me state right up front that I believe there is no connection whatsoever between hypnosis and what some people call paranormal activity. However, it is necessary to address this misconception since there must be some historical reason that it remains a public discussion. Let us define some important terms here.

The term *paranormal* refers to events or other phenomena such as clairvoyance or telekinesis that simply works beyond our understanding, scientific or otherwise. Clairvoyance is not a lady's name; it is the supposed ability to perceive things or events beyond our normal sensory contact. Some might use the terms Extrasensory Perception (ESP), sixth sense, or telepathy. Telekinesis is the power to move objects mentally or by means other than the physical.

In the infant stage of hypnosis development, particularly the eighteenth and nineteenth centuries, during the era of snake oil salesmen and other traveling charlatans, the publicity of the research into hypnosis caught the attention of performers and entertainers. Soon, hucksters roamed the countryside with rather wild claims, usually of one person being able to control some unusually gifted person into doing some incredible paranormal act. These acts would involve something like moving an object with his mind, reading a book through a brick wall, or some other fantastic performance. The problem was that none of these claims could stand scientific testing or review. Like today's TV faith healers, such acts may have made for good circus side shows, but there was simply no basis in fact to their claims. Any link to hypnotism is unfortunate because it now rests on hypnotherapists like me to debunk yet another misconception.

20. A hypnotist can make people commit immoral or illegal acts (or moral and legal acts). Here we are faced with basically the same problem that we addressed in #18 above: the hypnotist acting as a controller and the subject becoming a robot awaiting commands. The hypothesis is that one person can act like a drone pilot in control of another person who is acting as the drone. That is simply not possible.

We now understand this about hypnosis: First, hypnosis is a cooperative act between two people. Second, a person must have a fairly high level of trust in a therapist to even initiate hypnosis. Third, the subject is relaxed, but he is by no means unconscious. Fourth, the subject is highly focused on what is taking place; he understands every word spoken by the hypnotist. Fifth, the subject always controls his actions at that time and in the future. Sixth, a person under hypnotism cannot be forced to do anything against his will. Therefore, one cannot make another commit a crime or an immoral act unwillingly. Unfortunately, the opposite is true, as well. A person, against his will, cannot be made to give up a life of crime. If this were the case, we could do a bit of hypnotherapy and clean out the prisons!

To say this all in another way: hypnosis is not a tool that

can make a sinner out of saints, nor saints out of sinners.

21. Hypnosis in un-Christian, a tool of the Devil, and a play toy of the occult. This topic is so important to me personally that I have decided to devote the entire next chapter to its discussion.

CHAPTER 14

HYPNOTHERAPY AND THE CHRISTIAN FAITH

In our society which grows more secular every day, a culture that theologians now describe as post-Christian, you may wonder at the inclusion of such a distinctively focused chapter on a particular religious faith. The fact that I live and practice in one of the most multi-cultural communities in the United States may cause you further confusion at my taking time to pen this chapter. My marketing friends may be mumbling that I am breaking that old adage about avoiding the subjects of religion and politics in conversation.

Let me ask you to indulge me on this topic, though, and I certainly understand if you skip ahead in the book – this chapter is not a building block to the theme of the book. There are, however, several reasons for its inclusion.

First, when I initially considered hypnotherapy for my behavioral changes, I wanted assurance that I was not compromising my faith. I do not think that I had ever read an article or heard a sermon that specifically condemned hypnosis.

Nor does Scripture speak to hypnosis as we know it today, as it does against seers, soothsayers, and astrologers. It may be that I, with my lack of knowledge and understanding of hypnotherapy simply lumped the practice in with these biblically-condemned practices.

Christianity defines the idea of legalism as making something a sin that the Bible does not declare as sinful. In retrospect, I believe that is what I had done, even though I had never taken the time to logically consider my thought processes concerning hypnosis and its usefulness. Before submitting to the hypnosis, I needed to assure myself that I would not be dancing with the Devil nor dabbling in the occult.

Second, if you too are a follower of Christ or of some other faith, you may have the same questions that I had. Does the practice of hypnotherapy in any way counter the teaching of your religion? If so, maybe my journey will be of value to you.

Third, we often condemn those things that we do not understand. As I put hypnotherapy into context, I may be able to help you check your initial gut reactions against hypnotherapy and make a more reasoned consideration of the practice. For the most part, I will be "preaching to the choir" here. While this section will be of value to all readers, I write with my Christian brothers and sisters in mind, particularly.

If I were a Christian coming to this chapter, my first question would be "What qualifies this author to even address this issue?" The second question would be, "Doesn't he bring a bias to the discussion born of his profession and his need to make a living?" Both questions are fair and reasonable.

Please notice that my name on the cover is not followed by

a Th.D, a D.Min, a D.Div. or anything else that indicates an educated, professional prowess. I am not a seminarian, nor an ordained minister. I hold no formal degrees in Bible or in ministry; however, I am not devoid of any authority to address these issues. As the apostle Paul found it necessary to set out his credentials to the Philippians and to the Jews (Phil 3:4-6), I too will share with you my faith credentials, but not because I find it necessary. I realize that my works are but "filthy rags," and that my righteousness is found only in the gracious act of Jesus Christ.

As the old gospel song states, "I am just a sinner saved by grace." Raised by a devout mother, I professed my faith as a young fellow, and I have never looked back. In college, I began the discipline of daily Bible reading which I continue today. I have read the Bible cover to cover innumerable times (well in excess of fifty times, I would estimate). Today, my practice is to read five chapters each day, three from the Old Testament and two from the New Testament. For those keeping score, that gets me through the Bible about one and one half times each year.

I have supplemented my Bible reading with many of the great works of the Christian faith, including Augustine's *Confessions*, Luther's *Bondage of the Will*, and Calvin's *Institutes of the Christian Religion* (yes, all four volumes). Other favorites include works by or about Charles Spurgeon, William Carey, Jonathan Edwards, R.C. Sproul, John Piper, John MacArthur, J.C. Packer, John Wesley, George Whitfield, John Bunyan, John Newton, William Wilberforce, Billy Graham, and so many more.

It has been my pleasure to serve in many different

positions in many churches. I have taught Sunday School, served on local committees, and participated on the national board of the nation's largest Protestant denomination. I have served as the chairman of a private Christian school, on the board of a women's resource center, and in the local huddle of the Fellowship of Christian Athletes. Years ago, I was ordained as a deacon.

As part of my service, I made sure I was saturated with sermons, both written and oral, lectures, articles, books, podcasts, and videos on the Christian faith. I wanted to serve God knowledgably, intelligently and in accordance with His word. In Christian lingo, I am an inerrantist.

With such a background as mine, many would understand why I default to skepticism when I am presented with foreign ideas. Maybe it is simply a good built-in defense mechanism that makes me move cautiously when confronted with new ideas. When that cautiousness was coupled with loads of misconceptions produced by the entertainment industry and by media misinformation, I defaulted to skepticism about hypnosis and hypnotherapy, mixed with a healthy dose of mistrust, reactions particularly strong in the Christian community today. So, what are the roots of such a distrust of the practice of hypnosis?

What follows is a quick sketch of the diverse historical roots of hypnosis and hypnotherapy that have confused Christian believers and non-believers alike. Most major scientific ideas, like gravity or astronomy, developed around one person, such as Galileo, Newton, or Einstein. We can pinpoint a distinct starting point that leads to a paradigm shift for the scientific community. Hypnosis, as we discussed early, has multicultural roots. First, observations of the effects of hypnosis that have been happening for ages are now more readily understood. Second, what we now know as internal subconscious changes had been noted, but the causations of these changes have been debated over centuries. Cracking the code on the particular power of each person's mind, therefore, became not only a serious debate for the wise, knowledgeable, and scientific, but also a party for fools, charlatans, egotists, and religious devotees of various stripes. The mixing of science, opinion, and profiteering has been a recipe for a confused public. Such convolutions exist with the developments of many advances in science, but it is most pronounced in hypnosis.

While not an exhaustive explanation, we can see three major channels of development in hypnosis that have made hypnosis ripe for misunderstanding. In hypnosis, the results were predominate, rather than the cause. Therefore, people saw a wide range of behavioral changes, ranging from healed ailments, to attitude changes, to blocked or eliminated pain (as in hypnotic anesthesia). These changes were mystifying, and the debates centered on developing and controlling the skills to manipulate the changes.

One channel of thought theorized that physical forces outside the body could be manipulated to change what was interpreted as a mechanical device inside the body. At various times, people hailed magnetism as the key outside power. They argued that a body had two poles, and that a person with problems had his magnetism out of alignment. Passing a magnetic rod or other object over a person's body would help align a person's magnetism and help to bring about a cure. Fluidists made similar claims about body fluids being out of sorts. Developments in the understanding of electricity were naturally incorporated into treatments, as well. Some used physical touch to manipulate the physical nature of the inward problem. Various combinations of the applications of all of these outside manipulations added to the confusion of hypnosis.

A second channel of development focused on the operator (scientist, doctor, priest, or therapist) as the source of the subject's behavioral changes. When studies determined that such physical outside tools, such as magnetism or electricity, were not essential to the changes, people determined that the changes must be tied to the hypnotic operator. Again, such an explanation still leaves the impetus for the change outside of the subject. These operators varied in their interpretation of what would actually work to change behavior. Some claimed for themselves extraordinary and unusual skills or gifts, an especially good talent to have if you are trying to make a living. Another school of thought advocated strong demonstrative and authoritative control of the operator over the subject as the key. These people would demand or order the changes or cures to occur in the subject. Of course, these gifts and acts of dominance could easily blend together.

The third channel seems most related to our discussion of faith. In this group, people believed in neither external mechanisms such as magnetism, nor believed in the operators' gifts or authorities as key to change. This particular theory seems to originate with religious practitioners who attributed people's healings or transformations to deities or rituals. So, practitioners of witchcraft claimed their bewitching ways were at work, as did the occultists. Within Christendom, priests, monks, and early faith healers attributed the blessings to the Holy Ghost. Whatever the religious affiliation, early hypnosis-like activity could be attributed to the spiritual realm.

As expected, all three channels of development could easily become entwined over time. Therefore, we could end up with a monk authoritatively using magnetism and giving God all the glory for any success (and possibly blaming the sinner for any failures!). Such a range of claims could lead only to a wide range of scandals, reports of amazing failures and abuses, and scientific analyses that damned the science and stunted the hypnosis advancement. What kept the progress going throughout the challenges and catastrophes was that real, remarkable, and verifiable results of otherwise unexplainable healings and changes were occurring.

Slowly, from all of these divergent paths, the essence of the real transformations began to dovetail. Almost grudgingly, the focus turned from magnets, operators, and spirits toward the subjects themselves. What did the successful subjects have in common? In time, observers identified the trust and confidence of the subject both in the process and in the therapist as the first critical step. While some might attribute this trust to a belief or faith element, studies showed that successful hypnosis needs only enough confidence to create true cooperation between hypnotist and subject.

That understanding of the critical aspect of trust led to the realization that the mechanism for true change actually occurs within the subject. The individual's mind could do the heavy lifting in altering behavior. How that exactly works might still generate debate today, but the process is much like a complex computer. We have learned how to structure and input the data with hypnosis, but it is the Middle Mind that configures the data for change.

In time, researchers realized the importance of relaxation in enabling subjects to enter into productive hypnotic trances. Contrary to early practitioners who tried to drive subjects to a high level of excitement manifested by convulsions or seizure-like states, therapists in time learned that quiet calmness is essential for effective hypnosis.

In addition to the ideas of internality and relaxation, researchers also fine-tuned their assumptions concerning suggestibility. Suggestions are the form of data that the Middle Mind uses for processing. Trust plus relaxation and trance plus suggestion became the key formula to what would eventually become the successful science of hypnotherapy. Therapists also discovered an additional element, at least where permanent change is concerned: repetition. Once change enters the Middle Mind, that change needs to be solidified through repetition.

This winding road toward a successful formula for hypnotherapy, however, has left the public somewhat confused. Just as the new science of psychology found resistance among the public in general and the religious leadership in particular, the resistance to hypnosis stonewalled major progress. With the confusion and the fear of the unknown combined with the strange notion of "getting into someone's head," reluctance to embrace the practice is somewhat understandable.

The objection from Christians to the use of hypnosis, particularly as a therapeutic tool for good, are unfounded. There is a general belief among certain sectors of the church as a whole that a stance against hypnosis is official, which is not the case at all. The objections raised against hypnosis are not well-defined, but most seem to be centered on the prohibitions of submitting to forces other than God.

There is a sense in the Christian faith that we are to live righteously, relying on our own good sense as endowed by the Creator, and when faced with issues beyond our control, to prayerfully submit those burdens to God. Such a practice is actually a good one! The question arises, though, that if we are faced with a challenge and help is readily available, say an aspirin for a headache, a dentist for a toothache, or a heart surgeon for a blocked artery, can a Christian use these man-made resources? For nearly all, except perhaps the Christian Scientists, the answer is yes. So why is hypnotherapy not granted the same leeway? It must be the mixed message regarding the practice historically. Yet, hypnosis, despite its history, is moving into the mainstream, and as we embrace advances in medical treatments, it follows that we will embrace advances in psychology, as well.

Because hypnotherapy has proven to be so effective, we should embrace it as we have other medical advances. If we can alleviate the struggle of one child who suffers from a debilitating phobia, why should we not do so? Understanding what we do now about the therapeutic advantages of hypnosis, would we not be remiss in offering help to a fellow believer whose health is threatened by a life of obesity or smoking or drinking?

For centuries, Christian scholars have embraced treatments that help to heal people's suffering. No less than Thomas Aquinas (1225 – 1274) in addressing hypnosis stated that "the loss of reason is not a sin in itself, but only by reason of the act by which one is deprived of reason. If the act which deprives one of his use of reason is licit in itself and is done for a just cause, there is no sin; if no just cause is present, it must be a venial sin." The Roman Catholic Church in 1847 decreed that "having removed all misconception, foretelling of the future, explicit or implicit in vocation of the devil, the use of [hypnosis] is indeed merely an act of making use of [means] that are otherwise licit and hence it is not formally forbidden . . ." In short, the use of hypnosis as a tool for a just cause is not forbidden nor sinful. Reasonable Protestant scholars clearly agree.

Such a defense, however, does not suggest a Christian is to push the sovereign Lord to the side. As with all daily activities, the Christian must find his way to God, seeking guidance, wisdom, and protection. I certainly did while entertaining the idea of hypnotherapy for myself. It is the same as if I were facing medical or dental treatment or if I had a business or personal decision to make. Of course, every time I see a picture of myself now and see how much weight I lost or experience how healthy I feel these days, I cannot help but offer a prayer of thanksgiving for hypnotherapy, knowing what it has meant to me. My prayer now is that God will use me as I provide hypnotherapy assistance to others.

Even through the teetering years of hypnotherapy's development, some Christian leaders recognized the validity of the practice. In America, some of the most famous and earliest practitioners were ministers. In Great Britain, no less than Samuel Wilberforce, bishop of Oxford, examined the practice closely and encouraged believers to learn and practice hypnosis therapy in order to balance a field being dominated (and abused) by nonbelievers.

Most faith-based objections appear to be tied to misconceptions about hypnosis and the modern practice of hypnotherapy. Since those have been addressed in detail in prior chapters, they will not be rehashed here. But let us remember Robin Waterfield's words when addressing the misconception that a subject is surrendering his will to another during hypnosis: "Modern hypnotherapy is consensual, not authoritarian, and it is not the hypnotist's purpose to rob a patient of his will, but to channel his will power towards the therapy."

Where in the overall design of creation and in the history of man does the role of hypnotherapy actually fit? For the Christian, the overarching message we have is one of redemption through Christ for our sin that originated at the Fall. Besides the sin and separation that accompanied the Fall, we also bear the curse of living in a world that is sinful, broken, and under judgment. This state is manifested in many ways: man's cruelty to man, work that burdens and disappoints, disease that pains us physically, and ultimately death. While alive on this earth, we cope. When we are sick, we seek medicine or medical treatment. For other issues that come with life on this earth, we manage, employing help from others as necessary. Hypnotherapy deals with behaviors, and our behaviors are developed and programmed beginning with our first breath of life. Just as so much of this life is corrupted, so are our behaviors. For some, coping with stress becomes an issue. Others experience psychosomatic illnesses – real physical manifestations without an identifiable cause. Still others may have developed a trained response that limits skills or performances. The behavior that made me seek hypnotherapy was poor decision-making in response to food, eating both the wrong food and too much of it. In the perfect, natural state as God created, I would not have had these issues. However, as a fallen man, my Middle Mind is corrupt, and I am susceptible to self-destructive behavior. Hypnotherapy is a tool, simply one tool, that allows us to change some of these corrupt behaviors, or at least try to change them, in order to cope with the challenges brought on in the world. To deny this tool that has repeatedly been shown to be valuable in helping people is to deny a thirsty man a cup of water. The actual sin would be to deny fellow men the help that hypnotherapy provides. Those that deem it unchristian either misunderstand what hypnotherapy is or misunderstand what Scripture tells us.

CHAPTER 15

HYPNOSIS AND THE SCIENCE/MEDICAL COMMUNITY

I n 1543, shortly before his death, Copernicus published a work that challenged settled scientific conclusions. Until that time, it was a "fact" that the earth was the center of the universe. Copernicus postulated, rather, that the sun is the solar system's center, and that the earth orbited the sun. This new theory led to a war between the Church and scientists. It took six decades before the Roman Catholic Church took an official position against Copernicus' theory, which had started to gain traction, declaring it heretical. Over the centuries, other Christian communities also denied Copernicus' theory, widening the gulf between faith and science.

What history is slow to tell, however, it that science and the teachers of science who, up until then, were strictly geocentric (earth-centered) in their positions, caustically berated Copernicus and his views. Science, in lock step with the Church, also fought advances of the new idea. Science, like any other school of thought, is slow to accept challenges to its positions, fearing erosion of authority and position, and possibly profits, for holding the wrong ideas.

We have seen this same resistance throughout history. Joseph Lister pushed for more sanitary conditions and sterilizations in surgical and medical practices. The medical profession pooh-poohed his ideas, claiming such procedures were ridiculously time consuming and unnecessary. Untold millions world-wide died as medical providers dragged their collective feet in recognizing the truth of Lister's claims.

Although science is often hailed for innovations, true innovations that challenge entrenched and controlling ideas will always meet with resistance. The fact that hypnosis and its applications for treatment through hypnotherapy face such resistance should be expected. The resistance, to some degree, came from the Christian community. However, the challenges from the scientific and medical professions were no less pronounced.

Some of the debate is understandable. As we have already mentioned, in the development of hypnosis as therapy, it was difficult to identify the causal elements that led to success. No one wanted to debate the legitimate successful outcomes, and despite the fact that some of these outcomes were fraudulent and contrived, practitioners applied the scientific method to the results. They tested and reviewed the results. They analyzed data from the results, and they debated the data. If all of this work had taken place within the confines of a laboratory, it is doubtful that much would have been made of it all. However, hypnosis was a most public practice, made notable and irritating to the "establishment" in that the proponents of this new thing were a cavalcade of doctors, wisecrackers, preachers, charlatans, and profiteers. What a good show it must have been! No wonder the media have enjoyed reporting and caricaturizing it over the centuries. As convoluted as the progress has been, all healing professions have now accepted and even encouraged hypnosis for therapeutic applications.

Beginning in the late 19th century, hypnosis in general and hypnotherapy more specifically gained more acceptance and endorsements by professional associations and government agencies. In 1892, a special committee within the *British Medical Association* (BMA) investigated hypnosis. The report published in the *British Medical Journal* supported "the genuineness of the hypnotic state" and conclusively found effective use of hypnotherapy in "relieving pain, procuring sleep, and alleviating many ailments." Later that year at its annual meeting, the BMA unanimously endorsed the therapeutic use of hypnosis. That same report also marked as useless such ideas as magnetism, fluids, and other such historical speculations connected to hypnotherapy.

Again in 1955, the BMA made bold statements concerning the use of hypnosis in therapy. First, the *British Medical Journal* reported that hypnosis was effective in treating psychosomatic disorders, revealing previously unrecognized conflicts and motives, removing symptoms, changing morbid thoughts and behaviors, and relieving pain.

Then, in April of that year, the BMA approved the use of hypnosis in treating psychoneuroses and in hypnothesia for childbirth pain management and for surgery.

In 1956, Pope Pius XII approved the use of hypnosis for Roman Catholics, with these stipulations:

1. Hypnotism is a serious matter, not something in which to dabble.
2. Precautions provided by both service and morality must be followed.
3. When used as an anesthetic, the uses should be governed by the same rules used for other forms of anesthesia.

In 1958, the American Medical Association joined its colleagues across the ocean. Its Council on Medical Health not only approved hypnotherapy as orthodox medical treatment, but it recommended that training be included in medical school and encouraged additional research into the field.

In 1960, the American Psychological Association endorsed the field of hypnosis as a branch of psychology. It can actually be argued that the entire field of psychology finds its roots in the early developments and adventures of hypnotists.

1961 brought about more definitive guidelines from the AMA. Its Council of Mental Health specified 144 hours of training for medical students.

In 1995, The National Institute of Health reported that hypnosis is effective in alleviating chronic pain associated with cancer and other conditions, including irritable bowel syndrome and tension headaches.

In 2001, the British Psychological Society produced a report endorsing hypnosis as a proven therapeutic medium, beneficial in the treatment of a broad range of conditions and problems.

In 2003, the government of India through its Ministry of Health and Family Welfare endorsed hypnotherapy as a recommended form of therapy in India.

Today, according to the U. S. Department of Labor, a

hypnotherapist is one who "induces hypnotic states in clients to increase motivation or alter behavior patterns; consults with clients to determine the nature of problems; prepares clients to enter hypnotic states by explaining how hypnosis works and what clients will experience; tests subjects to determine degree of physical and emotional suggestibility; induces hypnotic states in clients using individualized methods and techniques of hypnosis based on interpretation of test results and analysis of clients' problems; may train clients in self-hypnosis."

Despite the early resistance, hypnotherapy is now uniformly accepted, endorsed, and encouraged by professionals in the medical and psychological field, as well as by official governmental agencies tasked with protecting the public welfare. Society as a whole continues to bring hypnotherapy into the mainstream of public acceptance and practice.

CHAPTER 16

YOUR FIRST HYPNOTHERAPY SESSION

So, you are contemplating hypnotherapy. You have an idea what your goal is. You know what problems you want to deal with, but the unknown about the process still leaves you a bit uncomfortable. Let's walk through your first session so that you will know what to expect.

The game plan for the first session has several goals, and those objectives will structure the appointment. First, the hypnotherapist wants you, the client, to be comfortable. Second, the therapist wants to build rapport and trust, an essential step toward success in the therapy and in the overall behavioral transformation. Trust encompasses more than just the idea of safety; it also contains the idea of confidence in the therapist and in his or her management of the partnership being formed between you two.

Third, the nature of your issue must be nailed down. It is essential to explore and diagnose the problem behavior that brought you to therapy in the first place. A key component may be the cause of the problem, and you can expect some discussions in order to help pinpoint the problem. However, hypnotherapy is a very progressive process, very future-oriented. Depending upon your particular challenge, the depth of cause examination may range from slight to substantial. For example, the origins of a smoking habit does not weigh heavily on the steps to behavioral change, but you should expect a question about how long you have been smoking.

Fourth, you will help set the outcome you want and the intermediate targets leading toward those outcomes. You would think that losing weight could include easily-defined targets. Not necessarily so. In my case, I entered into my first session thinking that losing forty to fifty pounds would be an amazing goal. I could not imagine returning to the weight I was in my twenties when I was running four to five miles daily. My hypnotherapist, Ken Thompson, thought otherwise. He encouraged me to shoot for a goal of eighty pounds of weight reduction. When I slipped passed the fifty pound loss mark, I realized the wisdom of my therapist. Being able to drop past the two hundred pound mark amazed me! As we (notice that I cannot help but refer to the team formed with my therapist) approached my agreed upon original goal of eighty pounds, Ken encouraged me to extend that goal to ninety pounds. Now we were talking about a weight that I had never seen as an adult, a weight that would take me back at least to my earliest high school years. As we hit the revised goal and adjusted my diet with a higher daily calorie count, incredibly my weight continued to drop. I felt like I was eating so much more food, but it was all good, nutritional calories, and my biology was happy with me and was showing me who I really was. Boom! There I was, one hundred pounds lighter and at a weight that I probably had not seen since junior high school. I had been an overweight child long before it was typical of school age children. I could not have imagined this result when I began my journey, but my hypnotherapist helped me to accurately define my outcome goals.

Fifth, once the targets are set, you and your therapist will set a schedule. The schedule includes the steps toward the goal, the progression of the therapy itself, and the timetable of all of the parts. At this point, if it has not already been established, the expected number of sessions for reaching the goals and forging them into permanent new behaviors will be set. Remember this, that no matter how many sessions are required, the speed at which hypnotherapy can achieve permanent behavior change is far faster than any other method of behavior change. Behavior change through chemical therapy or through will power rarely proves to be permanent and is often linked with health concerns (such as with the use of dangerous appetite suppressants or in the physical side effects of the Keto diet).

Upon your arrival, expect to find a quiet, comfortable setting. The therapist's objective is to put you at ease and create a quiet place that optimizes relaxation. This setting will be quite different from the bright lights of a physician's examination room. Hypnosis is not sleep, but the relaxation steps for the process present conditions very similar.

The hypnotherapist will engage you in conversations seeking to learn the information we have discussed above. One objective during this discussion, other than harvesting the key facts and developing the game plan, is to study how you communicate, both verbally and nonverbally. Do not worry about this evaluation; the therapist's goal is to be most effective in communicating well with you. Since the work is to take place in your Middle Mind, getting there needs to be in a language style that works for you, and then, while there, the suggestions that power your change must mirror your communication style.

In most circumstances, you will sit in a comfortable chair, maybe a recliner, and the therapist may or may not sit behind a desk. When it is time for the hypnosis section of the session, you might recline to assist with the relaxation. I found that I looked forward to each session. The discussion that took place, followed by a time of peaceful relaxation, was always rejuvenating and encouraging.

This encouragement is built in to the hypnotherapy process. Your Middle Mind is going to make the behavior change happen. The therapist wants to assist this effort by getting the right components for change communicated to your Middle Mind. Encouragement and positive reinforcement enhance and enable the process. Never fear good hypnotherapists. They are not belligerent task masters or hard-to-please parents. Rather, they are cheerleaders escorting you to success.

At the core of that success process is the hypnosis. As the session comes to a close, you will have your first entrance into hypnosis. There is absolutely nothing to be concerned about. As we discussed repeatedly, you are not asleep or unconscious, but you are totally aware of everything that is happening and in control of the proceeding. Your sessions work as a cooperative effort. The hypnotherapist brings a certain necessary expertise to the exercise, but you are the key.

Your number one job is to listen to the therapist. You will first go through what is technically called *induction*. This terms simply refers to the phase of the process that both relaxes you and helps you to narrow your focus. You might think of it as being similar to the quiet relaxation and thoughts that accompany you in falling asleep. In fact, the induction may very well make references to sleep, and if you are wondering how you can assist, just relax like it was nap time. Instead of pre-sleep thoughts of nap-time, though, simply listen to the therapist's voice. If your experience is like mine, you will be surprised at the lack of surprise. The surprise will hit you later as you experience subtle behavior transformations that change your life. You may not experience much the first time, it seems, except an encouraging period of relaxation. With each session, you will relax faster and deeper, and you will become more and more aware of the subtle, but effective process of hypnosis. Just enter session one with a positive intention to cooperate.

As you get more and more relaxed, the hypnotherapist will begin to implement the game plan for change. You will find much of your earlier discussions incorporated into suggestions that become the fuel with which the Middle Mind will operate.

As the hypnosis ends, the therapist will bring you out of the trance methodically so as to seal and reinforce the work accomplished during the hypnosis. With each session you will learn to relax more deeply, so that the end of the hypnosis may be akin to waking from a power nap. There is a refreshment that comes with the process.

The entire session will wrap up with final instructions. These may include homework of some kind, suggested items to observe for follow-up, and recordings of the hypnosis sessions you will use for reinforcement purposes. Do not let the phrase "homework" scare you. It will not be time-consuming like school work, but it is all necessary to the behavior change and the long term permanency that you want.

You may leave the first session with mixed feelings, an almost "Well, let's see what happens" outlook. That's what I did. With each succeeding session, I left feeling more and more confident, ready to conquer the world. May your journey be so, too, as you make your every day better.

CHAPTER 17

SELF-HYPNOSIS

U p until this point, hypnosis has been defined and demonstrated as a cooperative effort of two, implemented by the hypnotherapist and the client. But it is likely that you have heard the term *self-hypnosis*. Where exactly does self-hypnosis fit into the overall scheme of behavior change, though?

Chances are that as you have read this book, you have reflected on certain long term behaviors that you would like to change. Some of you may have even tested yourself, trying to make certain changes. It is possible that you have tried to will yourself into change. If you have a fear of heights, you may have intentionally made yourself ease to the ledge of a balcony. If you are a smoker, you may have sought behavior change with the patch or with nicotine gum.

Although I cannot discount that a person can, having never been hypnotized before, accomplish some form of hypnosis and ultimately some behavior change with some how-to books or maybe some CDs or videos, it is unlikely. Successful self-hypnosis is usually achieved in conjunction with standard hypnotherapy and the instruction of a therapist. Self-hypnosis and its uses and limitations are most understood by someone who has already had the benefit of being hypnotized multiple times by a professional.

When successfully used for major behavior changes, self-hypnosis becomes an adjunct to hypnotherapy, the objective being reinforcement and solidification of the gains made under the hypnotic trance induced by a trained hypnotist. There are several reasons for these limitations. For one thing, the depth of trances achieved in self-hypnosis is typically slight. As a result, goal achievements are limited. Secondly, suggestions, the making and communicating of the key components of change, are limited in quality and quantity. Some people recommend the use of a single suggestion, made over and over during self-hypnosis. Such a limited style of communication can reasonably be expected to slow progress, but this does not mean self-hypnosis is without value.

The problem we encounter in self-hypnosis is that the distance between our alert-thinking mind and our Middle Mind may confuse the process of self-hypnosis. We have to be alert and aware in order to guide ourselves into self-hypnosis, which is primarily a non-thinking process. We must both speak and listen to ourselves. The success in hypnosis comes with relaxation, the discharge of outside thoughts and considerations, and the single focus on the voice of the hypnotist. To be that voice, creating and issuing the suggestions, as well as the listening subject, conflicts with some basic tenants of hypnosis. As a result, the same gains simply cannot happen with self-hypnosis that can happen with normal hypnotherapy.

One of the requirements for any success with self-hypnosis is repetition; therefore a key component to successful hypnosis is the discipline to implement the program. You must be willing to set aside time regularly, which requires organizing your priorities. You will need to carefully coordinate work and family obligations so that your self-hypnosis is not squeezed out.

Finding the right location is another key consideration. A setting conducive to peaceful relaxation is essential. One of the benefits of seeing a hypnotherapist is the setting aside of time, leaving home and work obligations, and journeying to a place specifically designed to achieve your goals. If you are planning to use self-hypnosis at home, you will be well served if you can provide yourself with relaxing music similar to that which is usually introduced in hypnotherapy. Music serves many functions. It blocks out the everyday noises that surround us, such as the air conditioning, random building noises, chirping birds, lawn mowers, and such. But beyond that, music has been shown to stimulate different areas of the brain. While stimulating some, it calms and even suspends other areas of the brain. The right music need not be particularly entertaining, though. The goal is to find the music that works best for the Middle Mind to engage.

Once time and setting have been established, the steps to self-hypnosis will be familiar to anyone who has read the earlier sections of this book. The first step is induction, the process of reaching the hypnotic state. The primary goal at this stage is progressive relaxation. Relaxation will transport you out of the alert, thinking, day-to-day state of awareness so that you can dismiss the outside world, concerns, and thoughts. The body and mind must both relax. There are different methods of inducing relaxation and deepening the trance state. You will learn some of these patterns and suggestions from your hypnotherapist.

I must make a bit of a personal confession here. When I use self-hypnosis, as the relaxation process succeeds, it becomes more and more difficult to focus on the task at hand, even with the most simple and basic behavior change suggestions. Once I am relaxed, using the most pleasant imagery as part of my induction process, such as a quiet Caribbean beach or a mountain side stream in spring, I find myself enjoying the setting so much that it becomes a bit difficult to get to the next step, the work on the behavior change!

As an aside, if your goal is not truly self-hypnosis, but rather a time to withdraw from a hectic schedule and maybe catch a short 'power nap,' then the preliminary steps of self-hypnosis can help you achieve that goal even faster. Self-hypnosis can also help that common experience of the three a.m. wake-up that ushers in a flood of thoughts about work or family or that extensive to-do list that needs tending to, all of which make a return to sleep nearly impossible.

After achieving the deepest self-hypnosis trance possible - give yourself a heathy period of time to do this - it is time to move on to suggestions about your behavior. These suggestions should not be complex, preferably summarized within one sentence statements. They should address only one behavior change goal for each session. State them positively and in the present tense. Avoid any "I won't" or "I'm not" statements. For test taking anxiety, for example, you could say, "I have taken good notes and studied, and I know and recall this information at will." For a phobia of flying, you might say, "I know that flying is safe and fun, and it allows me to see the world in a pleasurable way." After slowly repeating your suggestion a number of times, follow up with some ego strengthening statements, proactive encouraging statements about yourself.

After almost fifteen minutes, it will be time to exit the trance. Likely, you will count your way out of the trance in a way similar to the method used in your hypnotherapy. During the induction process, you may want to include a suggestion about the duration of the self-hypnosis. It is uncanny what a good timekeeper the Middle Mind is!

Self-hypnosis is a very useful tool, particularly in partnership with standard hypnotherapy. If you attempt self-hypnosis without prior hypnotherapy and have little success, that in no way should hinder or color your evaluation of the effectiveness of hypnosis and hypnotherapy.

PART 3

MIDDLE MIND MAKEOVER – HYPNOTHERAPY AT WORK FOR YOU

CHAPTER 18

INTRODUCING APPLIED HYPNOTHERAPY

Part III of this book is designed to serve more as a reference guide to the various benefits that hypnotherapy offers. It is organized so that by simply scanning the chapter titles, you will have some sense of the breadth of applications and of the depth of the extraordinary, permanent, fast, healthy, and emotional benefits that many have achieved through hypnotherapy. As you scan the titles, you may see chapters that are of particular interest to you or that you may feel would be of value to a friend or family member.

I fear that often a list that claims so many benefits may actually give rise to a skepticism about the entire practice of hypnotherapy. Is this the modern snake oil that can cure all our ills? Or, even if the breadth of applications does not give you pause, maybe we have become too accustomed to seeing specialists for specific problems, such as in the medical field. For the cold or flu, the family practitioner is fine, but for something more serious, we look for a doctor who specializes in that particular organ or disease. "Maybe the family dentist is fine for a checkup or for a cavity filling, but I need an endodontist for this problem!" When you scan the contents of this section, you might be tempted to conclude that the hypnotherapist is overreaching her skill set.

Those are fair concerns, but hypnotherapy is different from other practices. The nature and mystery of hypnotherapy combined with how the Middle Mind works create quite a different dynamic than that of other fields. With the following subjects, the hero is you, or more specifically, your Middle Mind, rather than the clinician. Your incredible Middle Mind does the work. It receives the suggestions offered and in its own miraculous way and in fairly short order, it manipulates these inputs, modifying or "over-writing" prior habits, drives, instincts, or limitations with new behaviors.

So what is the role of the hypnotherapist and hypnotherapy? Think of it this way: If your Middle Mind were a computer, and your behavior were programmed software, then the hypnotherapist is the trained programmer, or more specifically, the trained re-programmer. The therapist first helps develop the new programming to be applied. Then he applies specific techniques to turn on the computer and to reach the "folder" for the behavior (in the Middle Mind). Finally, the therapist uses the right computer language for the Middle Mind. From there, your own internal operating system controls the re-write.

This nature of reprogramming allows one person to be involved in a broad array of hypnotherapy applications. To continue the computer analogy, suppose you had an idea for a new software program or for a modification of an existing one. You could employ a trained programmer to make it all happen. The programmer would need to know a bit about your current program and your objective or goal for the new or modified program. Then, in coordination with you, he develops the new program language. Basically, you are using the therapist to help you tell your own Middle Mind what changes need to be made in a language and with a method that will work for you. It is because a skilled therapist is trained in this general method of reprogramming that he may be able to help you, whatever your need may be.

The following chapters explain how general hypnotherapy techniques are applied to particular issues.

CHAPTER 19

PAIN

A. The Pain of Childbirth

Pain is often a warning sign of a physical injury. As such, a hypnotherapist typically wants a medical practitioner to examine the client to make sure that hypnotherapy for pain does not mask an ailment that needs serious treatment. That is not the case with childbirth, however. Everyone is familiar with childbirth to one degree or another. Since shortly after creation, most women have experienced excruciating pain during childbirth. Modern medicine has addressed the pain in several ways. For a time, most doctors administered general anesthesia. Now the localized relief from an epidural or other types of blocks is available for women looking to ease their severe discomfort.

Hypnotherapy, amazingly enough, offers an effective alternative to the chemical-laden medical intervention. The process involves two objectives: First, the relaxation and the therapeutic techniques prepare the mother emotionally and physically for the labor and delivery. Second, the hypnosis reduces or eliminates the pain during childbirth.

The hypnotherapist has several alternative approaches that he may use; all of them start with pre-labor sessions. The day of delivery is not the time to evaluate the mother as a subject of hypnosis or to introduce suggestions to deal with the discomfort. The early sessions will be learning times for the mother and the therapist. With each succeeding session of hypnosis, the mother's ability to relax and reach the adequate hypnotic level will improve. She will also be learning techniques of relaxation and self-hypnosis to use during the labor and delivery process.

The options differ, however, during the labor and delivery process, particularly regarding the presence of the hypnotherapist. One option is to have a hypnotherapist present at the time of labor and delivery, using her input to guide the hypnosis. The second option is to have the mother rely upon her earlier training in self-hypnosis during those pre-event sessions. Options vary depending upon the desires of the mother, the practices of the hypnotherapist, and the circumstances created and evaluated during the early sessions.

Reports from women who have used hypnosis during child birth are remarkably similar: a sense of relaxation, a lack of fear or anxiety, and some sense of comfort. Some have described a total lack of pain, while others describe a pain similar to having a monthly period. The mother experiences the physical aspects of child delivery, but without the intensity of the pain. Beyond the pain relief, women experience an incredible focus that attends the hypnosis. A mother is able to joyfully and fully experience the birth of her child.

If further medical procedures are required at or immediately after the birth, the attendant hypnotherapist can provide pain avoidance techniques at that time, as well.

Hypnotherapy can alleviate not only a wide array of a mother's post-birth conditions, including post-partum depression, the depression often experienced by new mothers, but it can also be useful for issues in raising children, such as bed wetting, thumb sucking, and ADHD. These topics are addressed later in Part III.

B. The Discomfort from Dentistry

Dealing with the pain of dentistry is our focus here, but the uses and benefits of hypnotherapy in this field extends well beyond pain control. The use of hypnosis in a trained expert's hands is so useful that dental practices in Great Britain employ full-time hypnotherapy practitioners in important support roles for treatments.

One important role of hypnotherapy involves those patients who experience anxiety or manifest absolute fear over dental visits. There is no one cause for this fear or anxiety. A bad experience, observation of other's fears, or just a person's own Middle Mind establishing a locked-in behavior from hearing and seeing stories in the media could initiate such a response. It is possible that the unfamiliarity in everyday life, the sheer "otherness" of dental operations and instruments and procedures lead to anxieties. Hypnotherapy has proven effective repeatedly both in reducing anxieties to moderate levels and in soothing fears and phobias about dental procedures. Because science has shown connections between many bodily issues and conditions originating in the mouth, concerns over drills and needles could lead to serious dental diseases or even greater problems without appropriate and timely interventions. Anxiety and phobias are addressed in more detail in another chapter in Part III.

In addition to alleviating anxiety and fear, a very practical use of hypnosis rightly applied is hypnothesia. Necessity has proven the value of hypnosis and bolstered its standing in the dental community. Just as wars of the nineteenth century demonstrated the effectiveness of hypnothesia for critical surgeries such as amputations (before the development of chemical anesthesia had really created a misplaced faith in pharmaceuticals), wars also contributed to a high regard for hypnosis in dentistry. The development of hypnosis for dentistry began in the prisoner of war camps of the twentieth century. The primitive conditions of the camps, the poor nutrition, and the lack of care, particularly the medical and dental care provided by the captors, led to serious dental challenges. Among the POWs were medics with some minimal dental training and, of course, actual dental professionals serving their countries. Dental decay and other oral problems became regular challenges. The POWs' jailers provided no care, generally showing utter disdain for their captives. This environment created the need for creativity among the prisoners, both in procuring instruments suitable for dental procedures, and in dealing with the pain of the procedures and of the post-operative healing. Hypnosis proved to be the answer! Before long, the use of hypnosis for relaxation and pain avoidance was commonplace among the prisoner camps. The success of the camp hypnosis treatment created a continued acceptance and of hypnosis throughout the war years.

With the end of war, however, the general focus of pain management shifted back to chemical agents for pain management. More recently, though, society has seen a modern war on pharmaceuticals, and hypnotherapy has once again proved useful in providing alternative for pain management. First, some people cannot tolerate chemical anesthesia, particularly if they are elderly or infirmed. Secondly, any use of chemical anesthetics comes with side effects and after effects, such as memory loss, dizziness, or nausea. We have all seen the hilarious videos of children and teenagers after oral surgery. Funny, right? Sure, but consider the danger or harm that such medication may produce. We can only speculate now, but with each passing year, we hear more and more how the pharmaceutical companies have profited to our regret. Third, post-surgical pain has led to what we now know can be a deadly reliance on manufactured pain killers.

Hypnotherapy provides the alternative to these dangers. The mind has an amazing strength and elasticity that can overcome many challenges we face; we just have to give it an opportunity. For the use of hypnotherapy for pain, I would suggest sessions with a hypnotherapist prior to the dental procedure in order to establish your comfort with the process. This session allows the therapist to measure the suggestibility as well as to discuss the anticipated dental procedure and the hypnosis process for the procedure.

On the day of the procedure you will be induced into an hypnotic trance. You will be awake and aware of your surroundings. You will be able to follow commands of the dental staff, but you will remain relaxed, probably experiencing a feeling of detachment and maybe even disinterest in what is taking place. You will be able to sense movement, but you will not feel the discomfort of the procedure. During this period of hypnosis, the hypnotherapist will prepare you for after care.

After dental procedures, patients may experience pain during the physical recovery. Hypnosis can be used to override any discomfort, and instructions in personal relaxations and self-hypnosis allows a patient to avoid any chemical dependency. Patients can expect not only to heal faster, but also to resume normal everyday activities quicker, too.

C. Phantom Pain (after amputation)

After an amputation, a patient in time may experience various forms of pain and other sensations coming from the site of the amputation. Sometimes it may simply be the feeling that the amputated limb is still present and functioning, but often it is a feeling ranging from discomfort to serious pain. The pain may be described as a shooting pain, and at other times it may be a stabbing pain, a cramping pain, or a burning sensation.

Typically, these phantom pains are associated with the loss of lower limbs, but the experience has also been reported with amputation of other appendages, such as with the removal of a breast, an ear, or a testicle. Even the removal of an organ can be connected to phantom pain. The appearance and degree of severity of pain vary among individuals.

Several theories exist on the causes of the phenomenon. One theory is that the severed nerves are trying to reconnect with the lost tissue, and these nerves sound the alarm of pain when the reconnection fails. Another theory believes the dysfunction lies within the peripheral nerve network. Some associate the dysfunction with the spinal cord, and others simply say it is a brain (mind) feedback system issue.

It is likely a brain feedback problem because hypnotherapy has proven so effective in managing the pain. Obviously, the function of naturally working limbs finds its automatic controls in the Middle (subconscious) Mind. With an amputation, the mind's programming has become confused and is struggling, even panicking. This confusion and panic is conveyed with pain. Persistent discomfort tells us the mind is not able to adjust and reprogram its network for messages related to the missing body part. The brain knows changes need to be made; it just does not know how to make them.

Hypnotherapy provides the method for the mind to resolve the issue. The Middle Mind is going to solve the problem, but it needs some informational input in order to do so. The steps of hypnotherapy act on several levels. First, the very process of hypnosis can produce greater relaxation for the client. This relaxation in itself can begin to provide some relief from the pain. Second, the suggestions "inputted" during the hypnosis becomes new data or programming that the Middle Mind can use to create new maps for handling signals from the site of the amputation.

An additional benefit from the hypnotherapy relates to the very emotional trauma associated with the loss of a body part. Often, these operations are due to severe accidents or to serious diseases. In either case, a person experiences emotional upheavals before and during the amputation process. The aftermath of dealing with the loss creates whole new sets of mental and emotional challenges in addition to the physical challenges. All of these experiences combine to create forms of anxiety and depression. Some might use Post-traumatic Stress Disorder (PTSD) to describe the situation. Hypnotherapy offers the tools to deal with these issues, as well. We will discuss these anxiety issues in more detail in later sections of this book.

Because hypnotherapy includes broad applications in dealing with phantom pain, it becomes the perfect tool to help those suffering with the issue.

D. Fibromyalgia Relief

As many as one in fifty people develop a condition known as fibromyalgia. Women are seven times more likely to fall victim to this problem than men. Onset is generally between the ages of twenty and fifty-five. As many as five million Americans have fibromyalgia. The name comes from three words: *Algia* for pain; *My* referring to the muscle; *Fibro* for tissues such as ligaments and tendons. With symptoms that go beyond just pain, sufferers refer to their fibromyalgia syndrome. Hypnotherapy seems to be reasonably successful in treating the pain associated with fibromyalgia.

Those suffering from fibromyalgia report an abundance of issues. Topping the list of symptoms are muscle pain, fatigue, and tenderness. Tiredness during the day can increase after the expenditure of little effort. After a day of fighting fatigue, a night of solid sleep would be welcome, but many sufferers report sleep issues, as well. Upon awakening, sufferers often report unexplained muscle soreness. The cycle repeats itself. With such physical issues, it is not surprising that anxiety and depression often follow. Irritable Bowel Syndrome (IBS) and Restless Leg Syndrome (RLS) will often accompany this devastating health challenge.

The cause of fibromyalgia remains a mystery today. Medical professionals will only identify a person suffering from this condition when they have ruled out every other possible physical cause. Having a formal diagnosis of fibromyalgia by a physician is a pre-requisite for an ethical hypnotherapist to treat a suffering client. The therapist needs to make sure the hypnotherapy does not mask a treatable physical ailment. Unfortunately for fibromyalgia clients, the condition is long term with a lifetime of health issues.

Since cause and cure remain mysteries, managing symptoms is the goal. Hypnotherapy has proven effective in test after test for reaching several key relief goals. The National Institute for Health states that of those suffering from fibromyalgia, those receiving hypnotherapy reported an outstanding 89% fewer pain symptoms. The study also noted that sufferers experienced fewer sleep problems, decreased morning fatigue, and decreased overall muscle pain.

With such physical results, anxiety and depression can be expected to decrease, as well. This change would naturally occur, but as we discussed in Part II, the hypnotherapy augments these results with therapy specifically for anxiety and depression. No wonder fibromyalgia sufferers report with joy the success of their hypnotherapy.

E. Complex Regional Pain Syndrome (CRPS)

Complex Regional Pain Syndrome (CRPS) is a rare but painful condition, one you may never have heard of. It is pain that develops in the arms or legs after a health challenge like an injury, surgery, heart attack, or stroke. Its cause is unknown, and there is no known cure. Besides the constant pain, which may last a lifetime, CRPS is considered a gateway illness, meaning that it may lead to serious even life-threatening problems, such as autoimmune diseases. Beyond the constant pain, CRPS can produce the expected stress, anxiety, and depression for its sufferers.

A hypnotherapist will require a formal medical diagnosis of CRPS before considering therapy, but hypnotherapy in conjunction with other medical care, such as physical therapy, has been scientifically proven to reduce symptoms, and in some cases, even achieve remission of CRPS.

Hypnotherapy allows a sufferers' Middle Mind to do its magic – reprogramming the autonomic nervous system (ANS). The ANS is the part of the central nervous system that handles actions we do not have to think about, such as stimulating digestion, checking levels of sugar in the blood, and regulating all internal organs. The ANS network can, when operating properly, use pain to warn us of issues that need our attention. With CRPS, the ANS is generating either an incorrect pain signal or one that cannot be interpreted, leaving the patient in agony. The hypnotherapist, through hypnosis, can help the client take new information in the proper form to the Middle Mind in a way that allows the mind to reprogram the ANS, offering some relief.

Of course, with this relief comes the additional benefit of less anxiety and stress, similar to what we noted with phantom pain and fibromyalgia.

F. Cancer, Surgery

One of the growing fields of study in hypnotherapy relates to the medical problems arising with our increasingly older population. We will focus this section on cancer, but many of the same principles apply to other serious diseases and surgical interventions, as well.

Just hearing the "C Word" brings waves of fear and uncertainty to diagnosed individuals and their loved ones. Some early diagnoses show immediately the stage and location of the cancer, enabling doctors to begin a clear course of treatment. In other cases, a diagnosis may only lead to additional testing, a lump to x-rays to biopsies to MRIs, with each step piling on emotional stressors. Treatments involve various combinations of radiation, chemotherapy, and surgery. Each of these produces its own sets of physical challenges, such as pain, nausea, sleep issues, and other bodily reactions.

Documented evidence of the effectiveness of pain control through clinical hypnosis shows the importance of this treatment for those faced with such a cruel diagnosis. Here are just a few:

- One study of breast cancer sufferers noted a schedule of treatment which included hypnotherapy demonstrated significantly lower pain and less increase in pain over extended periods.
- A bone cancer study concluded that those benefitting from the use of hypnosis had a significant overall

128

decrease in pain.

- Hypnotherapy was studied in a group of women with breast cancer who were having breast biopsies or lumpectomies. Against the findings of a control group that was offered empathetic encouragement, the hypnosis group showed significant decreases in the intensity of pain and in reduction in nausea, fatigue, and overall discomfort. Another group of women having large core breast biopsies using hypnosis reported reduced pain and anxiety, as well.

- The use of hypnosis with children undergoing cancer has also shown some effectiveness in helping with nausea and vomiting, debilitating problems particularly for children undergoing chemotherapy. With hypnosis, researchers found less anticipatory nausea and vomiting, and fewer overall issues with both nausea and vomiting throughout the chemotherapy. The researchers concluded that the changes brought through hypnosis affected both the thinking and the emotions of the patients. Other tests suggested that hypnosis also helped with nausea after surgery.

- Up to ninety percent of cancer patients report increased fatigue during chemotherapy or radiation treatments. Studies have shown that hypnosis intervention keeps fatigue from increasing during these treatments. Hot flashes in breast cancer survivors saw a seventy percent reduction in occurrences following sessions of hypnotherapy that included training in self-hypnosis.

- Sleep disorders also impact cancer patients, exacerbating their recovery. These patients report three times the insomnia as the general population. In one study, a set of five hypnotherapy sessions led to reports of significant improvements in sleep quality.

Before leaving the topic of cancer, let us look at how hypnotherapy works to help cancer sufferers, and what it can mean to those who have the worst of it, the terminal patient. Hypnosis can relieve pain and assist with related treatment issues, as we have seen with the previous studies. It accomplishes this feat in several ways. First, hypnosis with therapy can increase relaxation. Relaxation takes the edge off the pain, allows the patient to sleep better, and reduces the stress of the treatments, all which work to reduce anxiety and depression. Second, hypnosis may help to distract or dissociate the patient from the pain. Third, episodes of pain can seem to pass more quickly in the trance state, which serves to compress time. Fourth, the reduction in discomfort simply improves the entire treatment process as the battle with cancer goes on.

For those who are terminal, these benefits derived from hypnotherapy prove uniquely beneficial. Cancer is a most painful end of life experience. Currently, a person suffering in the final stages of cancer is increasingly chemically sedated for the pain. This sedation ultimately results in some level of dazed confusion; they may be with us bodily, but not mentally. Using hypnotherapy may allow a patient to remain alert and to enjoy his or her family right up until the end. Hypnotherapy allows a person's own mind to set aside the pain, creating a more peaceful transition from life.

CHAPTER 20

PERMANENT WEIGHT LOSS

I t is not news to anyone. America has a weight problem. The number of adult Americans considered obese is approaching forty percent, according to the National Institute of Health. Another thirty-four percent are considered overweight. So right at three out of every four adults in the United States are overweight, close to 200 million people. These numbers continue to increase. The next generations are going to be worse off, however, if current trends continue, as one-third of American children are considered overweight or obese.

The causes of this weight problem do not surprise anyone. We are eating too much of the wrong foods, and we are eating too little of the right foods – the clean, nutritional, healthy foods which (not surprisingly) are usually lower in calories. Regardless of whether we are eating healthy foods or not, we are consuming more calories daily than we should. It is that simple, and we know it. Culturally, we are more docile, inactive creatures, and as we gain weight, we move even less, putting on more weight and compounding the situation! I was the poster boy for modern America before my hypnotherapy.

Why are we like this? Why can we not change these trends? Because we have been (mis) programmed this way! We are not created this way. Our environment has certainly "shaped" us – round being our shape these days! It has influenced us through our Middle Minds. Our subconscious, but controlling minds, during critical stages of development have received too many wrong messages. It has been the comfort foods fed to us by parents. It has been watching friends in school as they munch those chips and drink those sodas. And the media certainly provided our little Middle Minds with images, sounds, and messages loaded with calories, from candies to sugary cereals to burgers and pizzas, colas and beer. Life's a party; let's celebrate and overeat all the wrong foods! Let's find comfort in bonbons or a tub of ice cream. And if you do not believe you have been programmed, think of the last time you had this thought: "I shouldn't eat this," and yet you did just that, probably within the last twenty-four hours. If not, your programming may be so locked in that you are past caring, at least until the next time you try to button your pants.

We know that this behavior and the attendant pounds do not come without consequences far more serious than just our clothes not fitting, however. The sheer breadth of health issues related to being overweight is amazingly sad. Being fat can lead to the development of Type 2 diabetes, heart disease (my issue) and stroke, many types of cancer, sleep apnea and other sleep disorders, osteoarthritis, fatty liver disease, kidney disease, and pregnancy problems. Emotionally, we are anxious, depressed, and despairing. Culture makes us want to hide – we simply do not look like the models and celebrities that fill the media, the John Candys and Chris Farleys being exceptions, and we do know what happened to them. Economically we suffer, as well. We are less active and less successful. We fail to get promotions. We lose sales because we are unattractive. Our emotions make us want to run and hide, not engage the world in a productive way.

America knows what it needs to do. We need to lose weight, and there is a $70 billion dollar diet industry (not including the fitness industry) out there to help us. Aren't we blessed?

Except there is a problem. Those pre-packaged meals, diet shakes, lite beers, calorie counting apps, color coded diet plans, weight loss pills and shots thrown in along with counseling simply do not work for most of us.

Ninety-five to ninety-seven percent of all diets fail. By fail, I mean that every study comes to the same conclusion: within one to five years, we will regain any weight lost during a diet , and often we add even more poundage on the rebound. Then the cycle starts all over again. We are certainly a nation of yo-yo dieters. I certainly was one. I had lost large amounts of weight, forty plus pounds, a number of times in my life. I soon learned that any weight loss was temporary, though. At first, I could fight the weight return for four or five years before the battle was lost again. With each subsequent diet, the "re-poundage" came a little quicker. At the end, I reached the "Oh, what's the use!" phase. I had reached the acceptance level of grieving.

Although I have had several semi-successful runs at weight loss, many were short-term diet failures, which, as it turns out, is also standard operating procedure for most Americans. The vast majority of diet attempts end within the first seventy-two hours. Nod your head if that has happened to you. What triggers these sudden failures? Consider the following scenario:

It is Monday morning, and you have committed to cutting back this week in order drop a few pounds. You weigh yourself, drink your coffee black, eschewing the sugar and the cream you prefer. You are off, having noted your weight first thing. Then you get to the office, and behold, Sam has dropped by everyone's favorite donut shop and brought in a dozen for the office. About mid-morning, someone sticks his head in your office and said it's Mary's birthday, and they are about to cut the cake. At lunch, there is an office meeting, and the meal is being catered – free sub sandwiches for everyone. That Lean Cuisine you brought with you remains in the fridge. The afternoon is spent choking down cups of coffee, trying to work through the various sugar highs and lows and the sleep-heavy feeling of that loaded meatball sub. Arrgh!

At least you can head home and have a salad, right? Tomorrow will be a different day. Maybe you can really make some dieting progress then. But home brings news of a sudden gathering of friends and neighbors. The home team is playing on national TV tonight, and the crowd is congregating at your place. Wings and pizza, chips and cookies, and ice cream are starting to arrive. And of course the beer is cooling in various ice chests being brought in.

So Monday was a disaster. The scales tell the story the next morning. Your excuse is that the sudden spikes in weight must be water retention caused by all the salt. Tuesday is going to be different. Ah, no doughnuts. Good. No birthdays, either. Are those hunger pangs you're feeling? What are the signals your body is giving you? You know your body is craving a sugar boost. Committed to fighting through today, you grab a glass of water and focus on the work at hand. The afternoon brings an email with a one day BOGO for your favorite Chinese restaurant. You fight the temptation. On the way home, you see that billboard with that mouth-watering burger displayed. You look away, only to notice every fast food restaurant along your route home. How do all of these places stay open!? You make it through Tuesday.

You fight the good fight all week. By Friday morning you swear the clothes are fitting a little better. You avoid Happy Hour with the gang after work that evening. Saturday morning brings good news. You are down a couple of pounds from Tuesday morning. Your spouse suggests a late breakfast at your favorite eatery. You tell yourself that you have been good. This will be your reward. And with that, all your effort is destroyed. The weekend turns into a nutritional disaster. Monday will bring a fresh start.

By Monday morning, the motivation is just not quite as strong. But you chug black coffee and head off for work. Then Sam rolls in with another dozen. Damn!

Why do diets fail? Our habits, drives, instincts are far too strong. They exist deep inside us – in our Middle Mind. They are much more powerful than anything our conscious effort and determined will can overcome. Our conscious mind and our will may push us through a day, or a week, or on very rare occasions toward a totally successful weight loss goal. For most of us, though, after some time all the weight returns, along with the despair.

To really lose weight and avoid fighting a losing battle the rest of your life, the core mental programming needs altering. This alteration is not a matter of the will. It is not a matter of education or re-education. Books won't help. Plans won't help. Apps will ultimately fail. Health coaches and pre-packaged meals are not going to get to the core issue – those ingrained behaviors that will rule the day.

The answer so many have been looking for, as it turns out, is incredibly effective, surprisingly fast, and best of all, permanent. Once the programming is set aright, the daily battles with the demon donuts and other temptations are effortlessly won. The answer is hypnotherapy.

In hypnotherapy those overwhelming drives that destroy your best dieting efforts can be "got at." That is the key: getting to the Middle Mind, where the worst habits and instincts subconsciously reside. That is step one. Hypnotherapists then provide clients with various tools they need to allow their own minds to effectively re-program to healthy settings. Literally, hypnosis addresses a lifetime of corrupted habits, removing and over-writing them with a new positive outlook and a winning plan for a lifetime of healthy nutrition.

The nuts and bolts of the hypnotherapy plan include the basics of weight loss: consuming fewer calories than you are burning. I use a basic, highly nutritional plan, and you can find everything you need at the grocery store. Regular monitoring of intake is essential. You will consistently measure your weight and review your progress.

I had the "terrible three" of the weight battle. I ate too many of the bad (high calorie) unhealthy foods. I ate too little of the good, nutritional foods, and I consumed too many calories total daily. As a client, I needed to first re-orient to new tastes and enjoy the good foods, like broccoli, which I now love. I needed aversion therapy related to sweets, fast foods, cheese and crackers, and so much more. I needed re-programming to better interpret signals from my body so as not to overeat. I am living proof of the subtle, almost unexplainable mind changes that can take place through hypnotherapy.

Your hypnotherapist needs to get to know you well, to identify your issues, and to coordinate your goals. With each session, you and your therapist will evaluate your progress and update your plan. Mixed in with the basics of the weight loss will be positive encouragement that will be a bonus of the hypnotherapy that sticks with you for a lifetime.

After you reach your weight goals, you will work to reinforce your new drives. As higher calorie-count menus are re-introduced into your daily fuel intake, you and your therapist will monitor and evaluate your new daily needs. As the sessions come to an end, you will be amazed at how your outlook on food and your dietary needs have changed. You will have tools and a new mindset to tackle the culture of overindulgence. You will have not only a new confidence that you have probably never enjoyed before, but also a very different perspective on who you really are physically.

CHAPTER 21

CONQUERING ANXIETY AND STRESS

T he vast majority of events that worry us never happen. Of those events that do happen, they hardly ever happen in the way that we anticipate. Yet, for many, these concerns cause us to agonize, and the anxiety results in emotional and physical stress.

Everyone experiences some level of anxiety. In fact, some anxiety at normal levels is necessary. Anxiety associated with emergency situations triggers the appropriate mental and physical responses. In normal day-to-day activities, anticipation moves us to action and production necessary for survival. However, anxiety that gets out of control severely impacts a person's life. It interferes with daily functions and eventually leads to long term mental and physical health issues. Anxiety combines feelings such as fear, restlessness, and worry, and it is often manifested in stress. Think of stress as everything opposed to relaxation. As with anxiety, some stress is welcomed. A gym workout involves intentional stress on our muscles. Normal work is accompanied by stress, such as getting up early in the morning and fighting commuter traffic. But stress triggered by unfounded anxiety can lead to heart palpitations, chest pain, digestive issues, and shortness of breath.

In fact, our physical health and physical acts point to stress brought on by anxiety. The list that follows highlights fifty symptoms of stress that can serve as warning signs that someone may need help. Hypnotherapy offers effective solutions for all of these.

- Frequent headaches, jaw clenching or pain
- Gritting, grinding teeth
- Stuttering or stammering
- Tremors, trembling of lips or hands
- Neck ache, back pain, muscle spasms
- Light headedness, faintness, dizziness
- Ringing, buzzing, "popping sounds"
- Frequent blushing, sweating
- Cold or sweaty hands or feet
- Dry mouth, problems swallowing
- Frequent colds, infections, herpes sores
- Rashes, itching, hives, goose bumps
- Insomnia, nightmares, disturbing dreams
- Difficulty concentrating, racing thoughts
- Trouble learning new information
- Difficulty making decisions
- Feeling overloaded or overwhelmed
- Frequent crying spells or suicidal thoughts
- Feelings of loneliness or worthlessness
- Little interest in appearance, punctuality
- Nervous habits, fidgeting, feet tapping
- Increased frustration, irritability, edginess
- Overreaction to petty annoyances

- Unexplained or frequent allergy attacks
- Heartburn, stomach pain, nausea
- Excess belching, flatulence
- Constipation, diarrhea, loss of control
- Difficulty breathing, frequent sighing
- Sudden attacks of life threatening panic
- Chest pain, palpitations, rapid pulse
- Frequent urination
- Diminished sexual desire or performance
- Excess anxiety, worry, guilt, nervousness
- Increased anger, frustration, hostility
- Depression, frequent or wild mood swings
- Increased or decreased appetite
- Forgetfulness, disorganization, confusion
- Increased number of minor accidents
- Obsessive or compulsive behavior
- Reduced work efficiency or productivity
- Lies or excuses to cover up poor work
- Rapid or mumbles speech
- Excessive defensiveness or suspiciousness
- Problems in communication, sharing
- Social withdrawal and isolation
- Constant tiredness, weakness, fatigue
- Frequent use of over-the-counter drugs
- Weight gain or loss without a diet
- Increases smoking, alcohol or drug use
- Excessive gambling or impulse buying

Some of the more common responses to anxiety include several areas that we will address with distinct chapters in this books:

Panic Attacks are sudden, intense periods of disabling fear. Often characterized by breathing difficulties, heart palpitations, and nausea, they reoccur unexpectedly, creating long term fear and anticipation of the next attack. We look more in detail at panic attacks in CHAPTER 25.

Obsessive thoughts are those undesired and repetitive fears on an idea or grouping of ideas provoking anxiety and disrupting life. Obsessive thoughts are covered in CHAPTER 25.

Phobias are a serious problem for many. Think FEAR. Not just any fear, or an appropriate fear, such as the fear of a rattlesnake you may have walked up on during your hike (run!), but an overwhelming and persistent fear of an object, a person, or a situation. Phobias often imprison a sufferer. We tackle phobias and fears in CHAPTER 25.

Low self-esteem is a problem for people with solidified poor (negative) views of themselves. Low self-esteem seriously handcuffs a person's entire life, affecting health, income, and relationships. Let's conquer low self-esteem in CHAPTER 38.

A variety of **digestive issues** from a run-of-the-mill stomach ache to a more serious and life-complicating disorder such as **Irritable Bowel Syndrome (IBS)** are caused by, linked to, or exacerbated by stress and anxiety. A closer study of these will be made in CHAPTER 28.

Sleep disorders, including insomnia, restless sleep, or limited sleep can all cause a lack of sleep that can contribute to other problems, including the problems of obesity, heart disease, diabetes, stroke, depression, arthritis, and kidney disease. Stress and anxiety are major causes of sleep issues, and we dig deeper into these challenges in the next chapter.

Hypnotherapists explore a range of particular themes during client sessions for anxiety. One early element of discovery involves the client's history with anxiety. The therapist will observe patterns of anxiety and stress, noting the effects of these conditions in the client's everyday life.

Another certain element included in therapy is one of encouragement, confidence building, and the raising of overall self-esteem. As a part of developing this positive outlook, the client and the therapist will discuss healthy, constructive ways of coping with legitimate concerns and will agree upon the implementation processes to make that happen. For instance, legitimate work concerns may lead to plans for seeking alternative work conditions or maybe venturing on to new employment.

The hypnotherapist will most likely assist the client in focusing on a constructive, realistic, but less worrisome future. This image will serve as encouragement in the present.

Elsewhere in this book, the processes of the actual hypnotherapy sessions are discussed in more detail. Hypnotherapy is both efficient in time and effective in results for those suffering with anxiety and the attendant stress.

CHAPTER 22

SLEEP ISSUES

A. Insomnia.

I nterrupted sleep patterns arise from a variety of causes: changes in the work schedule, sickness, travel schedule, a new bed. Insomnia - a broad term covering poor or inadequate sleep caused by difficulty in falling asleep, waking up frequently in the night, or rising too early - may be caused by a number of factors, but it only becomes a problem if it is recurrent over an extended period of time. For instance, once you have adjusted to that new bed, it may be time to examine other causes. Insomnia may be a result of many factors, some of which are just basic biology, others of the Middle Mind.

Your hypnotherapist will ask a number of questions initially in order to pinpoint the problem. Were there life events that coincided with the onset of the insomnia? What is your eating schedule like? (Eating too late can be a problem.) Are you consuming caffeine? When and how much? Are you ingesting other stimulants? What medications are you taking? What is actually contained in your supplement regimen? Do you use alcohol? Do you nap during the day? When and how much? The therapist will have practical advice regarding the sleep setting, the timing of daily activities, and the impact of your foods as he or she explores your habits.

Once these questions are addressed, the hypnotherapist will look at issues of anxiety and stress we mentioned in CHAPTER 21. Often, if insomnia proves to be anxiety-related (it very often has at least some component of anxiety involved), resolving the anxiety through hypnotherapy can correct the sleep issue.

Once the therapist has explored the history of the problem, she has a number of tools for use during hypnosis. Everyone understands how hard it is to try to think or will ourselves to sleep. The hypnotherapist may turn the tables on this "law of reverse" effect, the idea that the harder we try to do something, the more difficult it is.

The hypnotherapist may use techniques to help your mind ignore distractions such as street sounds, noisy clocks, or clicking ceiling fan.

A technique called dissociation may be involved in your session. Here, you will use the part of your mind associated with your problem to break down the "program" and change it.

Finally, the therapist will introduce the client to self-hypnosis. Here, clients are taught to take themselves to relaxed and near-sleep states of mind with just a few steps. Personally, I fall asleep easily at night. But if a power nap is called for, and I am a little too amped up, I can do a little self-hypnosis, quickly relaxing and boom! Forty winks, just like that – I am refreshed and ready to go.

B. Nightmares.

When I was a very young boy, my family watched an episode of a TV show called *The Outer Limits*. That night proved to be one of sheer terror for me. That still remains the worst nightmare of my entire life. The cause and effect connection being obvious, we never watched that show again, and my night of horror blessedly proved to be a one-and-done episode.

In the course of a lifetime, everyone expects a nightmare every now and then. Even if the cause is not obvious, nightmares are usually one night events. Others of us have repetitive dream plots, though they do not necessarily terrorize us. I have one theme that reappears in my dreams every year or so, one that I understand is a shared dream of many, of being in school again and being totally unprepared for testing in one subject. It is a weird dream to be sure, but it does not happen enough for me to worry about.

It is the persistent nightmare that needs attention. One that wakes you up, soaked in sweat, full of anxiety. The dream that really terrifies you. One that almost makes you fear to sleep again.

Hypnotherapy is effective for treating such nightmares. If a cause of the nightmare is not obvious from an initial interview, a therapist can use hypnotic techniques to search out potential causes, thus giving the client and the therapist the raw materials to build a plan for successful restoration of a good night's sleep. Once a cause is identified, if it is, it may open an entirely different toolbox of hypnotherapy approaches. Are there underlying health issues, emotional concerns, personal relationships, habits, or anxieties working their way into hours of sleep? If so, a therapist will address that particular issue directly during therapy, eradicating the nightmares.

The hypnotherapist can also structure therapies that provide the client's Middle Mind with the "facts" through direct suggestions to actually alter bad dreams so that they begin to tend toward more pleasant experiences. Even today, I am fascinated by the power in an individual's mind and its incredible ability to work effectively on its own, even when it is asleep.

A more advanced form of this Middle Mind control of dreaming is known as lucid dreaming. Although it takes some practice, lucid dreaming allows a client's mind to take a very active role in dreams. The script of a dream can be rewritten with plots changed, characters removed or altered, or the entire dream cancelled like a bad sitcom.

Hypnotherapy can sanitize those nights filled with nightmares, offering a more confident and peaceful sleep that gives a positive start to each day. And, as with all hypnotherapy, the success occurs rather quickly with accelerated behavior change.

C. Snoring

My son, Daniel, and I were looking forward to a father-son campout with a church group many years ago. Things went well until that first night. Most of the fathers were in two-man tents with their sons. Just as we began to settle into a peaceful sleep, this roar bellowed forth from one of the tents. A buddy of mine, a bank president no less, was shaking the trees with his snoring! Ah, the things you learn when you camp with buddies. He was sleeping, but no one else was. His poor son. His poor wife! It was the talk of the camp, and not in a positive way, the next morning. His response was a smile and a "Ah, that's just a sign of a clear conscience!"

Although a bit disturbing or a bit humorous, snoring can actually be the sign of a medical problem. Before consulting a hypnotherapist, a snorer should see a medical doctor to make sure that there is not a physical reason such as an obstruction that requires medical attention. Once physical causes are eliminated, a chronic snorer should seek the effective assistance of a hypnotherapist.

The hypnotherapist has several options to help lessen or even eliminate snoring; we will discuss four of them here. The first is a direct approach. The following three are behavioral changes that have the benefit of lessening the snoring problem.

Often snoring occurs when a person sleeps on his back. The airways of back sleepers are less open. This closure restricts air intake and the throat tissues vibrate, creating the snoring. Rolling to the side opens up the airway, thereby reducing or eliminating the vibration. Working with a hypnotherapist, clients can actually have their Middle Minds take control when they sleep. After a few sessions, the amazing human mind can learn to simply tell the body to turn to its side if it is on its back. This technique of hypnotherapy has been repeatedly used with great success.

Other factors, physically-related behavioral factors, that a hypnotherapist can alter with hypnosis to reduce snoring include problems with weight, smoking, and alcohol.

Because many overweight people experience breathing problems, they also have a greater chance of snoring. Reducing weight reduces the accumulation of fat around the neck and chest, opening the airway. Lose weight, reduce fat, and reduce snoring. It really is that simple for some. Hypnotherapy as detailed in CHAPTER 20 is an effective and efficient tool for weight loss to help control that snoring.

Smoking can also exacerbate snoring problems since it leads to the build-up of mucus in the airways and lungs. When a smoker stops the habit, mucus production is slowed, air flow is freer, and the snoring stops. Hypnotherapy is a reliable and effective means to stop smoking, as we will discuss in more detail in the next chapter.

Another culprit tied to snoring is alcohol consumption. Because alcohol is a type of anesthetic, it relaxes the muscles used in breathing a bit too much. A drink or two before bed sets up a night of snoring. Reducing alcohol or using hypnotherapy to alter one's consumption schedule are both possibilities with therapy. Altering this behavior curbs the snoring. For more detail on how hypnotherapy helps to treat alcoholism, see CHAPTER 33.

CHAPTER 23

SMOKING (AND VAPING)

Smoking

The economic costs of smoking are high. If a person smokes one pack a day, on average he will spend just over $2000 annually, according to the CDC. A two-pack habit doubles that amount to $4000 a year. Some statistics are higher, with a pack-a-day habit running to $5000 a year. But those are just the direct costs. What happens if the money spent on cigarettes were invested? And what about the accompanying medical costs to a smoker? A January 9, 2019, article in *The Atlanta Journal Constitution* actually reported that smoking in Georgia cost the least of all the states in the Union, but that the annual costs still came in at $27,390. In Connecticut, by comparison, that number jumped to almost $56,000.

Over forty-six million Americans smoke. Studies reveal that over seventy percent of those smokers want to quit, but as we all know, it is not easy to give up the habit. Ninety-five percent of smokers who attempt to quit will fail, and the cost of quitting is not much cheaper. A month's supply of nicotine gum runs almost $200, leaving the smoker still addicted to nicotine! The nicotine that naturally occurs in tobacco is as addictive as heroin and cocaine. As a stimulant, the cigarette offers an almost immediate buzz to its user. An adrenaline rush produces an increased heart rate, and a release of dopamine generates a pleasant feeling. Withdrawal is not comfortable, either, often accompanied by dizziness, headaches, insomnia, and general grouchiness.

The medical costs are well-known, too. Smokers suffer serious increases in the likelihood of heart attack, cancer, stroke, emphysema, and bronchitis. Second-hand smoke has been found to be a killer, as well. Family members of smokers are at higher risks for heart disease and cancer. The children of smokers have higher risks for middle ear diseases, respiratory infections, asthma, and middle ear infections. Low birth weight babies occur more frequently with mothers who smoke.

And then there are the social costs. A non-smoker not only lives a longer life, but it is a healthier, happier life. A non-smoker enjoys food more because it tastes and smells better. The clothes, car, home, and breath of smoker smell like stale smoke, a real turn-off to non-smokers. Smokers enjoy fewer employment opportunities, as well as job advancement opportunities. Their sports performance is decidedly poorer, and they spend much of their time worrying about quitting the habit. Not only will smoking lead to mouth and gum diseases, but it creates noticeably poorer skin tone and more wrinkles. Socially, it sets a bad example for impressionable children, who are more likely to become smokers themselves if they grow up around the habit.

Hypnotherapy is possibly the surest way to quit smoking permanently because smoking is both an addiction (to nicotine) and a habit. As tough as overcoming the addiction is, it is the habit that keeps bringing the cigarettes back. Hypnotherapy guides a smoker through detoxification and swiftly re-programs the smoker's Middle Mind, where all the habits are formed and stored. Because habits are learned behaviors that develop over prolonged time, they become virtually unbreakable without some type of extreme intervention, such as hypnotherapy. This therapy is key to permanently stopping smoking.

The list of habits vary from smoker to smoker, but they all know them. My dad told me of tapping his shirt pocket where he used to carry his pack of cigarettes years after he quit due to serious health issues. Others associate certain times in the day with smoking: over a cup of coffee; on the way to or from work; while reading a book or watching TV. To quit smoking does not mean we quit these activities, even though they have become triggers or indirect reminders of the habit. Hypnosis-based therapy gives the smoker the opportunity to break the power of these triggers.

If you are a smoker seeking a hypnotherapist for assistance in ending the habit, the order of business for the therapist is to get to know you and to explore the history of the smoking problem. He will ask a number of questions: why you want to quit, the extent of your habit (how many cigarettes you smoke each day, how many cigarettes you think or feel that you need daily), how many cigarettes you smoke simply out of habit, how the smoking affects your life, how you believe stopping the habit will benefit you, the age you began to smoke, what started your smoking, why you have not quit previously, or if you have, what precipitated your return to smoking, how much you spend on smoking and what are your plans for the savings, and finally, what fears you may have about smoking.

Fears about quitting the habit often hinder a smoker in seeking assistance. The hypnotherapist wants to flesh out those fears and make sure they are dealt with during the sessions. Addressing these fears is essential in making sure the client remains a non-smoker. A trained hypnotherapist is aware of those fears and knows how to address them.

Many fear gaining weight as they end the smoking habit. Hypnotherapy will provide the tools to make sure that will not happen. Many smokers see smoking as a way to relieve stress. The hypnotherapist is trained in helping clients deal with stress-inducing situations. What do I do with my hands when I am out with others, say at a bar? The hypnotherapist will use suggestions to help a client's mind instinctively handle such a situation. What do I do if I am offered a cigarette? You will have a plan and an attitude that helps you to easily overcome this situation. Finally, many smokers have a fear associated with the withdrawals that come with ending the addiction. The hypnotherapist will focus on strengthening confidence and resolve in order to cope with the discomfort associated with the process.

Quitting the smoking habit using hypnotherapy is a fairly short-term process, usually a matter of several weeks. My plan takes eight days. The key is that overall motivation and will power must come from the smoker's desire to quit.

Hypnotherapy is not magic, and it cannot overcome the client's contrary will. When I sought out hypnotherapy to lose weight, I was motivated by recent open-heart surgery that got my attention. Do not be the fool that I was. Get the right help before your health is threatened as seriously as mine was!

Vaping (e-cigarettes)

Vaping, a very plague upon our society, started with a noble objective – create a way to stop smoking, or at least to replace smoking with a less harmful activity. What it has created, however, is a harmful alternative and a crisis among young people. I suppose the developers were trying to limit the tar and many of the seven thousand chemicals inhaled through cigarettes. (For our purposes here, I am assuming no ulterior motives on the part of the original inventors.) Unfortunately, they wed a whole new set of chemicals and a dangerous delivery system to the evil nicotine, which remained the key component to an e-cigarette attraction.

In effect, the creators of the e-cigarette provided one bad habit to replace another bad habit. If there is any health gain at all, it is certainly a limited one. So far, vaping provides only a monetary benefit – it is less expensive than smoking - but in time that price gap may close.

Nicotine still remains a seriously addictive drug, and the vaper can increase the dosage by purchasing extra-strength cartridges for his e-cigarette. If you have read the prior section on smoking, you will understand that to quit smoking, you must overcome the nicotine addiction. The second prong of hypnotherapy deals with reprogramming habits. Vaping comes with its own set of habits, many of which are similar to smoking.

The real tragedy to me is the growing epidemic of vaping among young people. It was initially sold as an idea to teens as a harmless, fun, maybe even cool activity. Still, in many jurisdictions, there are no age restrictions on purchases such as those which apply to cigarettes. The lower costs also make the practice more readily available to youth. On top of all that, the purveyors of vaping began flavoring the product, broadening the market. For teens, nicotine alters and damages brain development, but for teens as well as adults, the harm to health is staggering, and, in its own way, comparable to smoking.

Health studies are just beginning to see the impact that vaping has upon the body. Vaping has been linked to cancer, and it damages the lungs, the heart, and the bladder. One dastardly ailment known as popcorn lung occurs when the smallest airways in the lungs are damaged, causing coughing and shortness of breath. Vaping increases heart attacks and alters the blood. It can damage the mouth, leading to gum and teeth problems. Recently, the combination of the vaporizer and the chemicals have been shown to damage skin, as well.

Friends and family are not immune to the hazards of vaping, either. As with second-hand smoke, second-hand vapor contains lead and other heavy metal particles that can harm those nearby.

The hypnotherapy process is very similar to the approach discussed with smoking. The hypnotherapist will need some background from the client on the vaping habit. The therapist and the vaper will solidify the objective of the therapy. I will especially be looking for the vaper's commitment to the process. The buy-in to quitting is essential to success. Most smokers seeking assistance are self-motivated. If the vaping client is a teen seeking help at a parent's suggestion or demand, the will power necessary to sustain the effort, an effort that truly is not overly burdensome, may not be present.

Hypnotherapy will include developing steps to help wean the client from the nicotine addiction, followed by the implementation of behavioral changes to address the habits that accompany practice. Finally, as with smoking, the client must deal with any fears he has. In the case of the vaper who uses e-cigarettes to end a tobacco habit, the therapist will work to prevent a return to smoking through hypnosis.

The sooner a person ends vaping, the better. We are just beginning to understand the health risks related to this practice. Current headlines of lung ailments leading to lung transplants indicate a frightful future for vapers. Hypnotherapy provides a successful and permanent method to squelch the habit.

CHAPTER 24

PERFORMANCE

This chapter will be a broad one, discussing topics from the bedroom, to the studio; from the stage, to the court; from the sales floor, to the course – whether golf or race. It may seem like we are lumping together too many diverse, unrelated activities. However, although the particularities of each activity may differ in execution, certain fundamental issues may hamper, to one extent or another, performances in each. Hypnotherapy provides an effective tool for overcoming obstacles and performing better. Using hypnosis as part of the process helps break through mental barriers formed in our Middle Minds. By breaking through these barriers, hypnotherapy can enhance anyone's successful performance.

Goal number one for hypnotherapy and for performance in general is to relax. We all, well, most of us, can carry a tune in the shower. In front of an audience is a different story, though. How does one move from the shower to the stage and still remain relaxed?

Closely connected with the ability to relax is a performer's confidence. Common to all performance activities is a need for confidence in one's self, one's skills, and one's preparations.

Focus, the ability to zero in on the objective when the bell rings, is another test for the performer. How to focus while remaining relaxed is always a challenge, but it is essential for success in all types of performances.

Most of us understand that to get better at any craft or sport takes practice. But practice for the more successful performers requires a certain amount of endurance or staying power that is beyond the average person. We have all seen coaches admonishing athletes to "dig deep," and we all sense that no matter how deep we dig, we could push ourselves just a little more. Hypnotherapy can be used to find that extra effort.

Finally, motivation overshadows the entire self-improvement goal in any performance. A person seeking hypnotherapy is certainly expressing a certain degree of motivation. The goal in hypnotherapy is to now channel that motivation into a more advanced level of performance.

A. Entertainment and Art

Acting. Hypnotherapy is perfect for actors who are encountering roadblocks to success or who are simply desiring to progress in their crafts to the next level. The very nature of acting makes this so.

Consider what an actor actually does. While the writer is the one who creates a person, fictionalized or based upon a real person, it is the actor who interprets the writer's intention on the stage or screen. Actors must be able to tap into their own emotions and knowledge of people in order to engage with the audience and create what the writer envisioned. If the role is based upon an historical character, the role is still an interpretation of the actor's in accord with the intention of the writer. To accomplish such a task, the actor must literally become someone else.

Such work requires creativity that is found within the Middle Mind (subconscious) where the instinctively creative and emotional aspects of the brain work. As the script is read, the Middle Mind takes the facts on paper and then gets to work. These creative "juices" of the mind are an awesome combination of God-given, innate gifts and life experiences full of emotions, instincts, drives, and habits. One goal of hypnotherapy is to make sure the actor can fully and confidently focus the Middle Mind on the task at hand, yet make sure the mind is free to fully explore and optimize the role. This "unbinding" of the mind takes us to the second aspect in which hypnotherapy can help.

Our Middle Minds have been programmed since birth. As a matter of survival and growth, fears, restrictions, and encumbrances have become almost hardwired into our personalities. A child growing up in a home with introverted parents can be expected to be less expressive herself. Parents and other influencers may demonstrate to us a need to temper our emotions, and we learn to keep them to ourselves. We develop our own personalities and ways of engaging with the world, and these modes of behavior become unconsciously applied in our daily lives. All of the encrypting of the Middle Mind becomes detrimental to an actor who needs to be free to express the behavior and emotions of a totally different person. The objective now is not to be his own person, but to be someone else entirely. Arguably, John Wayne simply played "John Wayne" in every role he undertook, and it worked for him, but that is not the limited range most actors shoot for. Just the other night, I watched Johnny Depp portray the mobster Whitey Bulger in the movie *Black Mass*. His personification of evil at times in the movie is far different from the lovable Jack Sparrow in *Pirates of the Caribbean*. What talent!

The hypnotherapist can assist the actor client with exploring the limitations to the development of his or her craft. Together they can formulate a plan that allows the actor's mind to be fed the raw materials necessary for the full development of creativity.

In addition to the creative nature of acting, the hypnotherapist can provide the tools to overcome other practical and individual challenges that actors face. Some of these may be issues that apply to non-actors, as well. Certainly, actors need to be comfortable as public speakers. They must not have stage fears or problems with performing in front of people. They need to be able to focus on their roles. They need to relax and yet to remember their lines and actions. They must have the skills to work with fellow actors. All of these individualized challenges can be unearthed and examined rather quickly. With hypnosis and suggestions, the actor's Middle Mind is empowered to re-create itself in order to overcome prior limiting behavior, replacing it with new acting-friendly strengths.

Hypnotherapy should be a consideration for any actor

wanting to improve, whether for a role at the local playhouse or on the big screen.

Singing. When it comes to hypnotherapy and performance, we all must start with the realization that we are not dealing with magic. We are talking simply about removing roadblocks to doing a task well. For a basketball player, hypnotherapy cannot transform someone who is 5′6″ into a seven footer. For a singer, hypnotherapy cannot create the talent; there must be some level of basic talent with which to work. My goal as a hypnotherapist is to empower the singer-client to better learn and exhibit his or her existing talent publically.

As with most performance-based issues, a core component of the hypnotherapy is getting control over anxiety. The anxiety comes from the evaluation that the performance will garner, whether it will be a test grade, a golf score, or public adulation (or criticism). In one sense, the performer should receive some pleasure simply from the exercise of the talent alone, but the desire to share the talent recognizes that judgment in some form lies ahead.

We must always remember that some anxiety is necessary. Pre-performance butterflies in the stomach have a certain benefit – they help get the necessary adrenaline flowing. Anxiety pushes some of the necessary buttons required for success in performances. However, anxiety can also cause the performer to tighten up. At an extreme, the anxiety reaches such a level that the performer completely eschews the public. We must wonder how many great talents the world has never experienced due to this phenomenon. We are all stars in the shower, but few want to try the stage!

So the goal becomes balancing the "good" anxiety with relaxation. How do we find that level of "shower performance" and move it confidently to the stage? That is the goal of hypnotherapy for the singer.

Anxiety usually manifests itself in several common ways. Singing is a technical enterprise, and as such, preparation is critical. Hypnosis can help to address the issues associated with incomplete or poor preparation, so that the singer can be more confident. Singers, like others, may focus on the negative feelings, becoming overly concerned with all the problems that can arise during a performance, dreading the response of the audience. This negative criticism from others and from themselves is one hurdle that therapy may need to address. Another roadblock to a singer's success is the intruding memory of prior poor performances. Therapy offers opportunities to overcome such hurdles.

As with any hypnotherapy, we would do well to remind ourselves that there is more than hypnosis involved in our therapy. So, as in any therapy, the therapist needs the client's history. For the singer, the therapist will want a brief but thorough recap of the performer's career up to that point. With the history, the therapist will be able to narrow the focus of the challenges that the singer faces. Working with the client, the therapist will set goals and determine the appropriate methods of hypnotherapy that best addresses them. The hypnotherapist will then script the therapy, including the use of hypnosis and post-session steps the client will implement.

Among other elements that may be a part of the therapy plan, a singer can expect to develop steps to address proper preparation. The singer will visualize future successful performances, creating a sense of encouragement for what lies ahead. He or she will learn to turn self-doubt and negative self-talk into positive self-communication and confidence. This confidence from hypnotherapy will be the key and overarching result of the whole process.

A singer who utilizes hypnotherapy will have an increased awareness of the changes she is making in her performance. She will be more aware of her surroundings and her talents. She will be more confident and relaxed, enjoying to a greater extent the talent with which she has been blessed.

Creativity: Art and Writing. Artistic endeavors and writing are included with the performance categories, even though they seem less public than other activities discussed here. However, these people who work with the creative arts experience many of the same general behavioral hindrances that performers face. Hypnotherapy provides the tools to unleash new depths of creativity, motivate new actions (overcoming writer's block, for example), and generate new, bold creativity.

As with all performance activities, works of the artist and the writer are for public consumption. Both know that their work is going to be judged by the public. Challenges with self-doubt, embarrassment, prior bad experiences (the art pieces that did not sell, the "can't miss" best seller that didn't sell) can all stem the creative juices and stymie the motivation to plug away. As life and all of its distractions hit, an artist or a writer may lose focus, leaving large gaps in the work at hand. How is one to push through, remain creative, and overcome the negative feelings? Hypnotherapy can provide the answer, and, for the creative sort, offer unique and truly appropriate remedies.

It has been estimated that we use about twelve percent of our brains for thinking, within our alert, working brains, that is. However, stored in the other eighty-eight percent of the brain are fully operating and accessible, through hypnosis, emotions, feelings, and memories, full of creative and brilliant ideas. Artists and writers have known for years that new worlds of creativity are within their own minds. How to access those worlds and free them for use has been the issue. As hypnosis has become more understood, many artists and writers have used it as the key first step to accessing the deep creativity of their minds.

As a hypnotherapist, my first goal is to get to know the client. What is his or her history as an artist or as a writer? What works has she produced and what successes and failures has she experienced? What motivates the artist? What is hindering her passions now? What are the sources of her inspiration?

After looking to the past and to the present, we now want to turn to the future. What are the goals that the artist or the writer wants to achieve? What are the hopes and aspirations? What fears accompany these desires? During all of these discussions, I want to get a sense of the client's confidence, motivation, persistence, and love of the craft. With this information, we now have the tools to make the necessary behavioral changes that will result in creative and confident progress. Together with the client, the hypnotherapist can develop the plan for the sessions, using hypnosis to allow the client's own Middle Mind to achieve the desired changes and to free the creative juices while providing encouragement and motivation to attack the work. The therapist will provide the tools for the client to work on post-session exercises in order to continue the progress begun in the sessions. Depending upon the circumstances, these post-session exercises may include reviewing session recordings and practicing self-hypnosis to be used in connection with the overall plan of success.

B. Sports

Golf. If I asked you to list the greatest golfers of all time, I bet that Jack Nicklaus and Tiger Woods would make your list. They should; they each have won more major tournaments than any other golfer in history. I doubt Tiger will catch Jack in the number of major tournaments won, but he certainly could. Besides being maybe the two best ever (being in Georgia, we must not forget the great Bobby Jones, though!), Jack and Tiger have another connection. They are both big believers in using hypnotherapy to improve their performance on the course. Tiger first began seeing a hypnotherapist at age thirteen.

Why hypnotherapy for golf? Golf can be a frustrating game to master. Any golfer has probably experienced the irritation of four hours of wasted time in a poor round of golf, one that leaves a golfer ready to chunk the clubs in the nearest lake. I once had a friend jokingly advise me to "Take two weeks off from golf . . . then give up the game!" What a character, that guy! Hitting a little round ball with a mallet and making it fly straight and long is difficult. It takes concentration, coordination, and in a full round of golf, a certain amount of endurance. To become skilled at the game takes a dogged persistence. There is enough pleasure in the game to keep many folks returning to the course, but it is an enterprise full of potential disappointment. If you have never seen the great Robin William's explanation of the origins of golf, give yourself a treat and watch this video now; you will thank me: *Robin Williams on Golf* at https://youtu.be/fui7yvebIdk.

Hypnotherapy provides help to the golfer across many aspects of the game. Utilizing hypnosis lets the golfer's own Middle Mind work to improve his or her golf game in many ways.

First, as with all performance activities, the golfer will develop a newfound confidence. The confidence will in time become much more than just a quick benefit. It will become a permanent change in the golfer's game.

Through hypnotherapy, a golfer can reduce anxiety about performance. As we have discussed elsewhere, some minimum level of anxiety is necessary to stimulate activity, but the self-control of such anxiety is essential to a good golf game.

Another advancement a golfer will enjoy through hypnotherapy is the ability to visualize individual shots and to mentally walk through a perfect round of golf.

The golfer will also learn to relax and quiet his mind. The ability to be relaxed and to ignore external distractions is essential to hitting that clear, crisp shot.

The hypnotherapist will assist the golfer in establishing a trigger or mental switch that he can flip instantly to reach the level of focus necessary to perform at the highest level.

Finally, hypnotherapy will help to create in the golfer the innate persistence to practice, to prepare, and to keep going in his pursuit of a better game.

The ultimate goal is for the golfer to enjoy a round of relaxing golf, leaving the course satisfied and ready to return again.

Tennis. Jimmy Connors used hypnosis-based training and therapy before winning the United States Open. Tennis greats Billie Jean King and Andre Agassi are both on the record as using hypnosis to help their games. Tennis hypnotherapy helps players to manage the multiple challenges they face during a match.

It is sometimes said that returning the hard serve in tennis is one of the most difficult challenges in all of sports. In this pressure-packed act, a player who is returning a serve must be alert, reactive, anticipating, and instinctive. Tennis, probably better than many other activities, epitomizes the cooperation between the conscious mind and what I call the Middle Mind (the subconscious). Hypnotherapy can first help a tennis player to relax. A tense tennis player is probably one who is counting too much on her "thinking" mind to succeed. While thinking about her moves or her structure, her feet become heavy, and the serve whizzes by. All the practice and the preparation are wasted in frozen thought. Hypnotherapy provides the capability to wed the super-focused mind with very relaxed and ultra-responsive agility. And that makes the game fun!

Let's look at some of the goals that tennis hypnotherapy can help athletes achieve. With any performance activity, the objective of the hypnotherapist is to use sessions to build up the participant's confidence. One of the amazing side effects of hypnotherapy is the encouragement and positive energy the client receives. Even if clients are seeking help with their tennis games, they will notice the overall positive impact in other areas of life, as well. Confidence is not just an in-game benefit. Confidence pervades the whole tennis regiment, from stretching to practice, to warm-ups to game-set-and-match, to match review and recovery.

In addition to confidence building, a leading benefit of hypnotherapy for the tennis player is the increased ability to focus under the twin burdens of pressure and fatigue. As an individual sport, tennis players are fully exposed. The success is individual, but so is the agony of defeat. The score evaluates the game, but so do the competitors and everyone else who is watching. All those evaluators build pressure. The pressure adds to the fatigue that comes with physical exertion of a most strenuous game. There is also a certain loss in concentration that occurs with fatigue. The ability to have the Middle Mind prepared to take over late in the match when the legs are rubbery and the conscious mind is weary will certainly lead to more winning shots on the court.

Hypnotherapy can also provide the player with new levels of endurance, both in the game and during practice. We all know we have a depth of reserve strength that we cannot seem to fully tap. Just as we will discuss in the section on marathon running, that additional push is available to the hypnotherapy client. Once a player has worked through and tapped into that endurance during game preparation, the strength and the ability to push through carries over into winning games.

Hypnotherapy builds up the bounce-back attitude needed for tennis players to exert the maximum amount of energy for the whole match. Players may make those embarrassing unforced errors and lose points, but a winner cannot dwell on a lost point. That bad shot is followed up with the next serve – right now! A successful player cannot let a lost point cost her the next point, as well. The attitude and ability to immediately reflect upon the cause of the lost point and add that information in a useful way to memory banks for spontaneous recall is entirely the function of the Middle Mind's super-consciousness. Enhancing this ability is a function of hypnotherapy.

All the components of a successful game coalesce in the Middle Mind. The Middle Mind needs to be programmed with a player's winning routine that becomes reaction, not thought. Anticipation of an opponent's actions must be instinctive. Timing and automatic responses and strategies are housed in the Middle Mind, and all these elements are encapsulated in a player who is calm and relaxed.

The advantages that hypnotherapy produces become obvious when the complex demands resting on a tennis player are broken down and reviewed.

Marathon Running and Triathlons. People involved in physical strength and endurance building have several similarities. One is a deep, deep feeling that "I could have done better" or "I know that I'm not achieving my maximum," yet despite their strongest endeavors, the signals from their bodies triumph over their minds. It is the weightlifter who fails to finish the set or fails to get up the extra weight. For the runner or the triathlete, it is falling short in times, missing preparation goals, and not enjoying the experience, knowing deep down that she could have done better.

On the other hand, there are those days when the athlete feels as though she can accomplish everything! For the runner, the legs feel like those of a light-footed gazelle floating over the roads, as opposed to the days when those same legs feel like those of a lumbering elephant plodding heavily through mud. You know those days! You feel inspired and exceptionally strong. Why can't every day be that way? And when you have those days, you sense that it is more than a physical thing, that something in the mind is acting differently. How can you repeat that magic?

The research shows that the Middle Mind (the super-conscious) not only affects the body, but it actually dominates the body. Doubts, habits, instincts, and limitations about physical activities hide there in the Middle Mind, and the keys to dealing with these issues and achieving optimal performance also reside there. Hypnosis used properly within the structure of hypnotherapy is the key to an athlete's maximizing his performance.

I once heard someone say that he would start running when he saw runners smiling. Sometimes, I think runners and triathletes do not enjoy their sport as much as they like simply overcoming or pushing through the pain to say, maybe only to themselves, "I did it." The act itself does not bring joy. The runner actually dreads each run. He knows that the pain is coming. The runner will "will" his way through it just to check the box. Hypnotherapy offers the tools to dump the dread, to create a positive outlook, and to anticipate every day as one of those exceptional days when the body is moving like a well-oiled machine, the feet feel lighter, and the whole experience is a joy.

Hypnotherapy is by its very nature an encouraging endeavor. It creates in all of its participants a positive outlook, and this is certainly the case for marathoners and triathletes. True, hypnotherapy is not magic. Its benefits do not appear instantly with the casting of a spell. Rather, the athlete should think of it as another form of training, with each exercise producing improved results.

Here is what you can expect in meeting with a therapist. The hypnotherapist will first want to explore your history with your sport. He wants to know your plans and goals. He will discuss your perceived obstacles to maximum success, as well as areas that you find are going well in your training and races. Now, together you and your therapist will develop a plan for your success in the Middle Mind training, right away taking steps to achieving those goals.

Depending upon the particular circumstances, some general goals for the sessions may include relaxation concerning the sport, a positive state of mind, a heightened endurance, a locked-in visualization of superior performance, training in affirming self-communication, and a built-in positive mental attitude toward the training schedule necessary to achieve your goals.

Triathletes face unique challenges due to the diversity of the events in this sport. For instance, a participant may have fears relating to open water swimming, or she may fear a bad spill on a bicycle, both of which could serve to hold performance in check. The hypnotherapist can provide the tools necessary to handle most of the unique issues that these athletes face.

The training is not exclusively at the hypnotherapist's office. The athlete will have tools and techniques that will accompany him to the practice track, as well as to race day. Athletes using hypnotherapy invariably show improvement. Runners not using hypnotherapy are likely not getting the most out of their potential.

Baseball. Pardon me while this author takes a little time to muse about his life-long love, baseball. From the Mighty Mites at age eight and through high school, baseball was my sport. This love is the reason I was thrilled to learn, as I first returned to the world of hypnotherapy, that many of the all-time greats of the sport have used hypnosis-based therapy to improve their games.

A brief roll-call of the stars who have used hypnotherapy makes my point: Rod Carew, Rick Gibson, Nolan Ryan, Steve Stone, Bill Buckner, Don Sutton, Mark McGuire, Maury Wills, Jim Eisenreich, Damion Easley, and John Smoltz. The Chicago White Sox in 1983 actually hired a team hypnotist and promptly made the play-offs. Just from this short list of players, we can discern a number of facts: The best players in the sport used hypnotherapy. Every player on the field can benefit from hypnotherapy, both the hitters and the pitchers. The effectiveness of hypnotherapy in baseball has been long recorded, going back at least to the 1960s.

Hypnotherapy is safe for all ages. Summit Hypnosis and Wellness (summithypnosisandwellness.com) records an ingenious Little League player who did his own research.

Working with a hypnotherapist, he determined that his on-base percentage increased by 15.5% after using hypnosis.

Baseball players have used hypnotherapy in a variety of different ways. Rod Carew, one of the most graceful players and best hitters of all times, first used hypnotherapy to overcome persistent pain after recovering from an injury. Jim Eisnreick had a problem with nervousness. John Smoltz, as a young pitcher for the Atlanta Braves, got off to an awful start early in his career in 1991. He sought the help of a hypnotherapist, turned his season around, and went on to a Hall of Fame career.

Each baseball player is going to have distinct challenges, and the hypnotherapy plans will vary based upon individual needs and goals. However, there are several objectives common to all baseball players.

My high school coach, a former St. Louis Cardinal, always told us that baseball was a "loosey-goosey" game. We all knew that meant that being relaxed was essential in playing baseball. Hypnotherapy is incredibly beneficial for players needing to relax and stay calm. But can being relaxed hurt a player when cat-like reactions are necessary? No. Being tense actually slows reactions. As we have learned throughout this text, relying primarily on our thinking, conscious mind slows us down. Focusing consciously on an objective actually brings the reverse consequences. The goal for every ball player is to prepare and rely on the Middle Mind, the subconscious, to take over and handle those immediate responses.

All athletes talk about being "in the zone," that mental state of highest performance. Such a state of mind is critical in baseball. Getting "in the zone" before taking the mound or stepping into the batter's box and then staying there is critical to optimal performance. In "the zone," a player experiences a high level of confidence combined with tremendous focus, but it is not a focus that is forced. It must be a focus occurring naturally, originating in the Middle Mind. Optimizing "the zone" is a unique accomplishment offered by hypnotherapy. A ball player will become adept at entering "the zone," a place where quick reactions and anticipation exist and where the crowd and other distractions are totally ignored.

Finally, a baseball player using hypnotherapy will have an enduring positive attitude. This confident attitude will persist through tedious practices, long road trips, and extra-inning games.

Although the focus of this article has been baseball, many, if not all, of the components apply to its sibling sport, softball, and to its cousin, cricket. (England's cricket captain, Mike Brearley made use of a sport hypnotherapist.) You can read a brief review of other sports for which hypnosis combined with therapy works well in the next section.

Other Sports. Hypnotherapy has such success in enhancing athletic performance because all sports share common attributes. Sports involve human-versus-human competition. Success in competition brings victory, and victory brings reward, even if it is nothing more than satisfaction of prevailing over another, or of seeing practice and preparation rewarded in the arena of competition. Typically, in one form or another, others are evaluating the efforts of sports performers, whether it is by the fans in the stands or the buddies in the clubhouse. Someone is always watching, or so we think. If nothing else, we are evaluating ourselves as we compete and often we are the most critical judges of our own performances.

So, although every sport has peculiarities that may distinguish the approaches that are taken in hypnotherapy, all share common needs. Athletes need confidence and the ability to relax, but at the same time, they must be highly focused and able to endure, even as the body physically objects. Athletes need to prepare and not procrastinate in their preparation. They need to enjoy their sport, for sports truly are meant for recreation. The real objective should not only be a trophy, but joy in the doing!

Since hypnotherapy has broad applications to performance improvement and has the flexibility for modification in different sports, it becomes an intricate part of every athlete's plan for success. Hypnotherapy has been successfully employed in a variety of sports. Besides the sports we have already discussed, the other sports where hypnotherapy has been applied successfully include:

- Alpine Skiing
- Auto Racing
- Basketball
- Body Building
- Bowling
- Boxing
- Cricket
- Cycling
- Diving
- Marksmanship/Competitive Shooting
- Mogul Skiing
- Pole Vaulting
- Rugby
- Shot Put
- Skeet Shooting
- Speed Skating
- Soccer
- Softball

- Figure Skating
- Free-Style Skating
- Football (and Futbol)
- Gymnastics
- Swimming
- Track
- Weightlifting
- Volleyball

C. Sales Performance

Sales Call Reluctance. For the non-salesperson, a career in sales does not look so very complicated. For those engaged in sales, however, the human-to-human interaction contains as many complexities as courtship or political diplomacy. Sales call reluctance involves a failure to prosper and a failure to self-promote. The causes are all emotional, deep-seated within the Middle Mind, practically hardwired into a struggling salesperson. It could be fear of the unknown or the fear of failure. It may be fear related to public speaking or interpersonal engagements. There may be reluctance to appear pushy or aggressive.

Only for the most unusual person in sales has one or more of such fears not caused a knot to form in the stomach at some point, or the heart to race, or perspiration to bead, or feet to drag. A battle rages within us between the need to succeed in making a living and the years of Middle Mind programming that seems to fight us along the way. We have read all the books, many which are "guaranteed" to show us the way to make sales easy and productive, and yet when the pressure is on, when the lights turn on and the bell rings, the same old emotional obstructions appear. Even as we push through such feelings, we know our reluctance limits our success.

Hypnotherapy provides the tools to efficiently change a

175

salesperson's entire perspective on work. Let's consider the steps in the hypnotherapy process for quickly overcoming sales reluctance.

Step one is to unearth the emotional roadblocks, the programming, the neural pathways that have taken a lifetime to form and which have been solid barriers to the salesperson's success and happiness. Some of these roadblocks may be apparent to the client, but he will need to examine and deal with even the most obvious obstructions. Other emotions that hamper success may not be as clear, but the hypnotherapist will be able to assist in the self-discovery process. In extreme cases, advanced techniques may be necessary during hypnosis to assist in hunting down and identifying the problem "programming" issues.

After identifying the issues, the client and therapist will deconstruct the components that created and reinforced these negative habits and influences over the years. These emotions are almost set in concrete. They may have taken years to develop and solidify, but hypnotherapy offers a shortcut to re-program or over-write these stultifying and previously uncontrollable emotions.

Once the therapist and the client have a picture of what habits, influences, or emotions are causing the problems, they will work together to establish the goals for the therapy. The client will identify what success looks like. What does the salesperson want to feel like? How does he want to feel? How does he want to act following hypnotherapy?

With this information, the hypnotherapist and the client can coordinate the overall plan for the sessions. With this roadmap, the client and the therapist can begin to make the necessary changes toward success.

As part of the plan, the client will have real, concrete activities in hand in order to practice new behaviors and habits. The salesperson will be able to implement these new behaviors in the prospecting and contacting of sales targets. Because there must be a way to test and measure a client's progress, the salesperson will report on the real life applications of the work he is doing during the hypnotherapy sessions. Such reports allow the "team" of therapist and client to re-visit every step in the program, from identifying root emotional causes and roadblocks to plan development and then to make any adjustments necessary. For weight loss clients, their calories still have to be counted and their weight measured, even though the ultimate key to weight loss is Middle Mind modification, since all weight gain is really related to emotional actions. With sales call reluctance, we measure sales production, and with each step in the progress, we measure whether the controlling emotions are changing.

The key step in making that change, the step that allows the entire process to move so rapidly, occurs during hypnosis. As we so thoroughly explored in Part II of this book, the hypnosis sessions allow clients, in conjunction with the therapists, to efficiently get at those deep Middle Mind issues and make the changes. Here the client's own Middle Mind is given the bits of information it needs, in the proper form, to do the work of "fixing things." The capabilities of a person's mind are extraordinary, and each client's mind, in its own way, will bend, reform, and readjust, all in incredibly creative ways. Also, during these sessions, the client will achieve on-going boosts of relaxation, confidence, and focus, the common "side-effects" of modern hypnotherapy. People seldom realize all the positive effects of the hypnotherapy process until they experience it for themselves.

In the final step, a client will apply all of the in-session effort to real world practice and to experience the success that has been missing. Together with the therapist, the client will follow up these real life applications in later sessions, with the goal to make all corrections permanent as rapidly as possible.

Procrastination. I have been meaning to write this section for some time, but I have been putting it off. Just kidding. But there are many who procrastinate so often that they face much of life with anticipated regret, and it is not a laughing matter.

Procrastination is simply delaying, postponing, or putting off action. It is a habit, and in those who struggle with it, procrastination is a very real problem, impacting regularly and negatively their lives. For the purpose of this book, I placed this topic under Performance since it definitely affects job performance and under Sales because the adverse impact of procrastination can be measured in dollars and cents for salespersons. However, procrastination can negatively impact far more than earning capacity, and these comments about how hypnotherapy can successfully help the procrastinator apply well beyond the business world.

Procrastination can lead to missed opportunities. It can create long hours at work, late work hours, and disruptions in time with friends and family. Work that does get done is frequently of lesser quality because it is rushed, which ultimately results in lower paying jobs, or in some cases, dismissal from a job. Around the house, relationships can suffer as spouses, children, and other family face repeated disappointment. People will learn not to trust a procrastinator, and eventually people will simply avoid one altogether. All of life can begin to crash in on procrastinators, as they are overwhelmed with incomplete projects, jobs, and obligations. Dreams die, and ambition turns to stress. Stress leads to a panoply of mental anguish and physical dysfunction.

The causes for procrastination are varied, and a client will need to explore these with the hypnotherapist. Ultimately, it probably finds its origin within man's natural aversion to work, but most of us overcome this innate inclination to avoid work as the drive to survive and thrive wins out. Many people actually enjoy work. In my case, I cannot imagine not working at something. Retirement is something of a foreign concept to me, as I always have this "I am just getting started" feeling. However, for many people, there is enough frustration with daily work that they battle regularly against their inclination to put off tasks. For some, in their Middle Minds, there was either a failure to create enough positive work habits, or a development of mental obstructions in dealing with tasks promptly, effectively, and efficiently. Procrastinators often lack confidence and have a tendency to overanalyze tasks, as well. In the earliest phase of hypnotherapy, the therapist and the client together will explore the particular circumstances of the client's issues. As with all cases of hypnotherapy, this discovery process is not a long, drawn-out process that takes weeks and weeks. Usually, a therapist can determine primary causes immediately, enough so that he can construct a plan with enough flexibility to be modified seamlessly during sessions.

Although each plan for success in overcoming procrastination will be customized for the client, common elements to each therapy session exist to help re-write the script of habits in the Middle Mind. Overcoming procrastination requires the formation of new, instinctive, and automatic responses when the client faces new tasks. A client will experience greater positives as she begins to see tasks as opportunities rather than burdens. She will take events that previously triggered habits of procrastination, and she will turn them into automatic triggers to implement new, more productive approaches to those events.

Sessions for procrastination will create an approach that develops a confident and relaxed response to new opportunities that were once seen as unbearable burdens. Relaxation is a precursor to so much that occurs during hypnotherapy. It is essential to the use of hypnosis, but it is also a continuing by-product of the hypnotherapy process. Those of us who experienced hypnotherapy for a particular need are continuously aware of how much more relaxed we are when we face all the events and challenges that life brings. Part of the relaxation is certainly a result of a growing self-confidence that results from hypnotherapy. Hypnotherapy, in practically all successful forms, is a very positive and encouraging process.

A successful plan for defeating procrastination is implemented in the hypnosis portion of the session. [CHAPTER 10 explains the mechanics of hypnosis.] The hypnosis will typically take ten to fifteen minutes, a relaxing time during which the client is fully aware of all that is going on. The goal of hypnosis is to give the client's Middle Mind the raw material (in words) that it needs, in the proper form, to allow it to do its own programming. As we have emphasized throughout this text, the individual's own Middle Mind is the real hero of hypnotherapy success.

When she returns to the real world, the client will have an approach in hand that she can apply to concrete situations. These real world interactions will become the basis for reflections and revision of the approach as she defeats her procrastination habits. Remember, the goal of hypnotherapy is not to simply fix the problem; it is to make sure that the fix is permanent. The first step in ending procrastination begins now. Don't delay. Act!

D. Public Speaking and Stuttering

Public Speaking. In an old comedy bit, Jerry Seinfeld refers to a study that showed that people are more afraid of speaking in public than they are of dying. He then jokes that at a funeral, the person giving the eulogy has a tougher job than the one at the center of attention. Some people truly feel that way. My wife is a former high school English teacher, and her experience shows that the fear of speaking publically starts young. On more than one occasion, a student was willing to take an F on an assignment rather than stand in front of the class. In business settings, such as networking events, I have seen the struggles of those who felt forced into public speaking because their jobs require it.

We place this issue under the Performance category since public speaking requires a certain degree of public performance, even if it is within a small group. Some people may not feel that they have a real fear of public speaking; they do not have sweaty palms or panic attacks. In fact, they may even enjoy it, but many people do feel that they need to improve the execution of their speaking.

For others, it really is a situation in which they may welcome death or some other tragedy rather than deal with the overwhelming anxiety and all of its physical and emotional ramifications of public speaking. For these sufferers, this article could appropriately be included under Phobias and Fears. I will address issues with public speaking here, recognizing that there are some links between basic execution of speaking publically and the outright fear of getting up in front of a group of people.

Fear of public speaking is not something born into us. It is a learned behavior, frozen within our Middle Minds. Often, it comes from personal traumatic experiences as children. Maybe it started when the teacher called on us to answer a question in class or to read orally in class, and our classmates laughed at our mistakes – oh, the natural cruelty found often in groups of children! It is possible the teacher offered no help or even reinforced the criticism. One of our natural desires is for approval, and such public embarrassment following a performance creates great awkwardness and guilt. Such emotions are building blocks for our undesirable future behavior. Some children unconsciously (maybe in tandem with conscious intent) never speak publically again. Most of us will continue to speak just fine to individuals or in small groups, but given a larger group or a more formal setting, we simply freeze.

Even without such frightful direct experiences, difficulties with public speaking can still set up shop in our Middle Minds. Observing fear of public speaking in our parents or siblings – important examples in a child's life – may demonstrate a behavior that will be subconsciously adopted. Early on in my life, I developed a pleasure in public speaking, mostly in association with leadership positions in school and on the ball field. My children were able to observe their dad enjoying the preparation and delivery of speeches, so that they too enjoy public engagements, one now working as a lawyer and the other as a teacher.

An even more subtle negative influence on our development as public speakers comes from the role everyone experiences as a listener to other's speeches. We evaluate and criticize. We compare notes. "Susie spoke poorly." "Josh must be embarrassed." We may see the problems of poor speaking at work in lackluster leaders or in school with boring teachers. One way to avoid being those teachers, leaders, Susies, or Joshes is to simply avoid being in their positions. This idea, tied to our negative emotions, becomes locked in our Middle Minds and our behaviors.

These fears become automatic thoughts, controlling thoughts. People cannot successfully will their way out of such thoughts. Even if they do manage to force their thoughts to change, their efforts may be poor, reinforcing prior problems.

For those who are not phobic about public speaking or who do not reach a level of anxiety typical of a phobia, but who still fail perform well, continued poor performances will negatively impact any future attempt at public speaking.

Hypnotherapy provides effective and speedy results. As

with all hypnotherapy, the therapist will need to briefly discuss the client's history and characterization of the problem. With the end goal of successful speaking always in view, the hypnotherapist and the client will examine more closely those pertinent areas that will need to be addressed. Depending upon the discoverability of causes or the severity of the speaking fear, further evaluation of past issues under hypnosis may be beneficial. The control of prior fears or issues may be an element of the hypnosis segment if those base instincts must be dislodged for progress. Otherwise, the hypnosis aspect of the therapy will be future-focused. However, such work is in no way unusual, difficult, or extensive. Relief from the fear is a beautiful thing!

Every client has different needs, but every plan that a client and therapist coordinate will certainly contain some basic elements. First, the plan will include methods to generate relaxation when preparing and delivering public talks. A Middle Mind predisposition toward relaxation in conjunction with techniques to create that relaxation will be objectives of the therapy.

Working hand in hand with the development of relaxation is the development of confidence. Confidence and vigor are by-products of any successful hypnotherapy, but they are a real focus for public speakers. Confidence is attractive and pleasing. It eliminates self-doubt and negative self-talk and oversees all preparation and delivery.

While important to public speaking, confidence and relaxation can work successfully only with solid preparation. If there are any hindrances to quality preparation, such as procrastination or poor focus, the therapist and the client must address those during hypnotherapy. A speaker who thoroughly understands his subject and who uses an organized approach will certainly create successful presentations.

It is one thing to give a speech. It is another thing to have something to say. Passion about the topic ties together the effective work of preparation with the need to please, impact, and persuade an audience. Hypnotherapy will help to knock down the mental barriers that sabotage the energy and passion that should naturally accompany any topic.

Persistence and practice are two important elements that any competent speaker needs. Not every sermon that preachers will preach create fire and motivate congregations, but they keep on preaching. Every speech is an opportunity to learn, improve, and perfect. Developing the habit of persistence will be a tenet of hypnotherapy for those seeking public speaking help. I have seen raw, fearful speakers in time turn into confident, engaging ones. Many with public speaking issues experience stunted skill development while avoiding the underlying issues. Recognition that catching up takes a little effort will be part of the hypnotherapy.

Soon negative thinking patterns will be a thing of the past. A group of cruel children will now be an audience of encouragement that needs to hear from you. Confidence, gained through hypnotherapy, will accompany you to the podium!

Stuttering and Stammering. Most people use the terms *stuttering* and *stammering* interchangeably, but others have characterized these issues somewhat differently. Some think of the word *stuttering* as more of an American word, with the word *stammering* as more British. Some professionals make a distinction between the two. One group labels stutterers as those with problems speaking the first part of words and stammerers as those having problems completing words. Still others say that stuttering refers to those who repeat the first letter of a word, such as s-s-s-sandbox, and stammering to those who simply get stuck at the beginning of every third or fourth word. Country music legend Mel Tillis would probably be labeled a stutterer under this latter distinction, while King George IV as portrayed in the award-winning movie *The King's Speech* would be a stammerer. For the purposes of this section and for application of hypnotherapy to the problem, we will treat the terms as synonyms. Being American, I will simply refer to the malady of stuttering.

Stuttering has one of two distinct origins, one successfully treatable with hypnotherapy. Stuttering for most of us is part of a developed behavior, usually created during childhood, but in rare cases it can develop later. For these cases, hypnotherapy is quite successful. However, stuttering can also be caused by physical reasons, such as brain trauma. I have a dear friend who has survived the removal of a huge benign brain tumor. He has been left battling aphasia, a condition that impairs his production of speech (as well as reading and comprehension of language). He might be thought to have a stuttering issue, but it is a bit more complicated than that. He simply cannot come up with the right word at the right time. His impairment is actually greater than that of a stutterer since the stutterer will know the right word, but he will just have problems saying it. I would suggest even people with physical issues, though, experiment with hypnotherapy to give their minds the opportunities to re-write some Middle Mind programming.

Hypnotherapy provides not only assistance in exploring the causes of a client's stuttering, but it provides the tools necessary to develop the plan for therapy and to execute the plan. Hypnotherapy has proved a consistent benefit to those seeking help for stuttering, sometimes with very public success stories. One of the most recognized voices of all time, the voice behind Darth Vader, was once a stuttering voice. James Earl Jones's use of hypnotherapy resolved a stuttering issue, leading to the voice we know today. Actor Bruce Willis also resolved a stuttering problem with hypnotherapy.

Everyone from time to time stutters. It is normal to occasionally have speech mix-ups due to searching for the right word or from getting distracted. But for most people these mini-challenges do not snowball into continuing problems. For stutterers, small matters lead to bigger difficulties, and these difficulties then move to the forefront of every attempt to speak.

The nature of the causes for the stuttering will direct the development of a client's hypnotherapy plan. The plan in hypnotherapy is always future-focused. The focus of therapy regarding root causes will vary. Once the issue of causation is addressed, therapy will turn to behavior-changing steps. These steps will no doubt include real world applications, reporting, and evaluations. The therapy will work to eliminate negative self-perception and negative self-talk and to instill the confidence and joy in communication that will enable speech to come easily and naturally, the way we were intended to speak. The process of hypnotherapy for clients dealing with stuttering is generally short-term, as compared to other forms of counseling and therapy. Multiple sessions will be necessary in order to confirm that the plan is succeeding and to make any adjustments necessary as the therapist and the client evaluate the progress. Remember, the goal of all hypnotherapy is permanent behavior change, so sessions will be scheduled so that permanent success is insured.

E. Test-Taking.

K-I-K-O, or Knowledge in - Knowledge out, explains the two focuses of hypnotherapy for those who underperform in test-taking. It is understandable why so many consider themselves poor test-takers. Testing by its very nature is pressure. It evaluates a person's performance, rendering our best efforts to a letter or a number. The fear of not measuring up and failing the evaluation overwhelms some who understand the short-term and long-term ramifications of the test, from advancement to the next grade, to admission into the "right" college, and ultimately toward future employment opportunities. Teachers evaluate. Parents set expectations and demands. Fellow students critique efforts. Although the simple K-I-K-O formula would seem to outline the path to success, Middle Mind emotions rise up to devastate many at exam time.

1. Knowledge-In. If a student is not prepared and does not have the knowledge necessary to pass the exam, all the positive attitudes and confidence in the world cannot help. Having a good knowledge base, on the other hand, contributes greatly to a proper test-taking attitude.

Hypnotherapy identifies problems with study habits that the client may have. Those problems will become the targets of behavioral change utilizing training, therapeutic counseling, and hypnosis. Not every client will have study problems, but for those who do, the hypnotherapy will need to address some or all of a number of issues. Many students put off studying until it is too late to prepare adequately. For those, a goal of hypnotherapy will be to stop procrastinating.

A student's lack of focus both in the preparation or in the test-taking itself may be a concern. The therapist will help the client to explore the causes of such a lack of focus and then work with the him to establish a plan, often involving the use of hypnosis. In conjunction with the improvement of focus, the therapist may also guide the client toward eliminating distractions.

Students with comprehension issues benefit from hypnotherapy, as well. During sessions, the therapist and the client will explore the nature and causes of ineffective comprehension. Once they have determined the barriers to effective comprehension, they will develop a plan to boost reading results.

What good is comprehension without retention, though? To that end, the hypnotherapist will tailor sessions, as well as out-of-therapy practice, to improve memory.

Poor time management and less-than-efficient study habits typically create poor test results. Regardless of the type of education, studying correctly and studying enough are essential to success. Together with the client, the hypnotherapist will be able to evaluate these habit and determine a solid plan for improving both the client's use of time and use of study techniques.

2. Knowledge Out. Now that the preparation work is done, let's work to get the student into an optimal position to perform at test time. The ultimate goal is a relaxed, positive, and confident test-taker. If the full material is comprehended and retained, test taking should be the celebration of the effort that was put in during study time. For many, however, test time can produce the horrors of anxiety, creating disastrous results. To make sure that does not happen, a hypnotherapy plan will first make sure that the student-client knows how to take a test that he has the basic test-taking skills and approaches to succeed. It is difficult not to excel if the student enters a test period with a plan and an approach for success in place.

The hypnotherapy plan will also address behaviors to optimize recall at test time. Part of the way to improve recall is to deal with anxiety, the real bugaboo of test-taking problems. Hypnotherapy is a tried-and-true way to learn to relax, to develop confidence, and to know how to peacefully "turn it on" for test taking. The hypnotherapist's goal is to ensure that the student has the tools necessary to get into a winning mental performance zone at test time.

F. Sexual Performance

Many men and women suffer from problems associated with sexual performance. Most of these problems can be treated effectively through hypnotherapy. However, a hypnotherapist should not begin sessions until a medical professional has ruled out any physical causes for the problems. For instance, even at young ages, as many as one in five men experience erectile dysfunction (ED), with that percentage increasing with age. Of those dealing ED, as many as twenty percent experience a psychological cause that hypnosis can treat. Only when the physical cause is eliminated should a person seek help with hypnotherapy.

Hypnotherapy for sexual performance is not just for men. Many women experience sexual dysfunction that is linked to emotional or behavioral development. In women, the issues may be vaginismus (painful tensing spasms of muscles during sex), frigidity, anorgasism (inability to achieve orgasm), or simply lack of sexual desire or drive. In addition to erectile dysfunction, men may also experience impotence, premature ejaculation, and a lack of sexual drive that may impair performance.

The causes for those problems vary as much as individuals themselves vary. Outside stressors, such as financial concerns, work turmoil, or family conflict can create performance obstructions. Anxiety, whether it is related to those stressors or just to the performance itself, can lower the sexual drive. Many times, these issues are related to past, often very normal, experiences that have generated Middle Mind (subconscious) behavior patterns that have become impossible to overcome. Other emotions such as guilt, in all of its various forms, and depression can lead to sexual dysfunction. These emotions can create low self-esteem, indifference, and a general apathy that can manifest problems in the bedroom. Hypnotherapy can address these emotions, thereby helping to increase a person's sexual performance.

In hypnotherapy, the therapist will work with the client to explore the root causes and to develop a plan of therapy that addresses those causes. Through hypnosis, the client will be given the tools necessary to change those emotions and, thus, the behavior.

The ultimate goal coming out of hypnotherapy is a client who is confident, encouraged, and positively anticipating the sexual experience. An eager anticipation of a very natural, intimate experience will replace the debilitating pressure to perform. Many people have enjoyed a more robust, intimate relationship with their significant others with hypnosis-based therapy.

CHAPTER 25

FEARS AND PHOBIAS

ll phobias are fears, but not all fears are phobias. Some fears are very healthy emotions, but phobias are not. A phobia is defined as an unhealthy, extreme, and irrational fear or aversion toward an object or situation. Thus, when people face the object of their fears, their behavior is outside the normal realm of reactions, despite the fact that they may actually understand the irrationality of their reactions.

All fears, with the exception of two, are learned. [Babies are born fearing only loud noises and falling backwards.] Most fears that we learn are healthy, as we learn to avoid death, injury, or pain. These fears are made instinctive in our Middle Mind as we grow and learn. Fear of being burned by fire or hot things in the kitchen is necessary. Fear of dangerous snakes is wise. Learning to fear falling from heights is a solid survival strategy. However, shrieking at a picture of a snake, or sweating profusely while riding an escalator, or avoiding a kitchen completely when the stove is on are illogical overreactions to fears that can impede lifestyles. A phobic cannot rationally change his or her reaction. Logic and reason do not reach the Middle Mind where these mis-programmed behaviors reside.

Anxiety always accompanies a phobia. Phobics recognize that their fears are unreasonable and their reactions are excessive, but they can only try to avoid the object of their fears. They cannot consciously overcome them. Depending upon the seriousness of the phobia, the trigger will vary. The fear of a diamondback rattlesnake is valid. Severe fear generated by a television video of a rattlesnake, however, rises to the level of a phobia. A still photo of a rattler which causes some type of anxiety is a more severe problem, but a fear generated simply by the mention of a rattlesnake is now reaching the extreme level of a phobia.

To be a phobia, a fear must elicit an irrational behavioral response. I do not like snakes of any kind. All snakes get my attention, but once I am comfortably far enough away to evaluate the type of snake I have encountered, I am reasonably calm. I have no need to scream, strike it, or faint unless it threatens me in some way. I am a big believer, though, in long handled shovels as my snake weapon of choice, should I need it.

A person who views a snake from a safe distance and yet breaks out into a sweat, even if the snake is not a threat, may be suffering from a phobia. A racing heart, shrieks of fear, and a furious flight may be next. At its worst, uncontrolled panic attacks and hyperventilation may overwhelm a phobic.

Phobias need attention when they begin to interfere with

normal lifetime activities or relationships. A fear of flying by a family member can impact the travel plans of the entire clan. Typically, one who suffers from a phobia understands his fear is unreasonable, and he may be embarrassed by his reactions. This embarrassment may lead to withdrawal, as even the acknowledgement of the fear becomes an object of avoidance.

Phobias can start in a number of ways. Remember, phobias are learned behaviors; they are not learned solely in the conscious mind. Facts may enter the mind, but our emotions are involved in constructing and cementing our fears. Sometimes a single traumatic (and emotional) event can trigger a phobia. A severe car accident may create a fear of driving or of even being a passenger in a car. A series of smaller but troubling events can also generate phobias such as the flight attendant who develops a fear of flying after repeated trips dealing with turbulence.

Stress of any kind can attach to something totally unrelated to the stressor and generate a phobia. A spouse experiencing stress in a marriage is more susceptible to developing a phobia. A student under stress may fixate upon something totally unrelated and become irrationally afraid of pencils. A child being physically disciplined by a parent can have an emotionally charged response to a certain location (closets, rooms) or objects (belts, shoes).

While some phobias develop through events that happen to us, others develop through events that happen to those around us. A mother who is afraid of spiders or mice is likely to influence the developing behaviors of her daughter. Those whom we most respect and trust may serve as examples in our lives to foster the development of phobias.

Most common phobias can fall into several broad categories. The first category, **Insect and Animal Phobias**, include the typical suspects (spiders) to the more docile (cows) and to most of the creatures of God's creation, both great and small. The second category, **Natural or Environmental Phobias**, include fears of darkness, heights, and water.

Medical Procedures and Injuries form a third category of phobias. Here we include the fears of receiving injections, having surgery, or dealing with any other type of medical, usually invasive, procedure.

Situational Phobias make up a relatively common group of fears that include fears of flying (aerophobia), enclosed spaces (claustrophobia), and open spaces (agoraphobia). Other less common situational phobias include fears of elevators, fears of escalators, and even fears of attending school.

There are some fears that defy categorizing. Where do we put Cosmo Kramer's fear of clowns? I recently read of a woman who used hypnotherapy to overcome fears related to all things "Michael Jackson." Apparently as a child she was traumatized upon viewing Jackson's *Thriller* video, and the fear had morphed into a fear of his music, his image, and of any reference to him at all. Another report stated that one woman suffered high levels of anxiety when she observed other people eating. What a recluse she became before benefitting from hypnosis-based therapy.

Here are the ten most common phobias, starting with the most common:

- Arachnophobia (spiders)
- Ophidiophobia (snakes)
- Acrophobia (heights)
- Agoraphobia (open spaces or crowded spaces)
- Cynophobia (dogs)
- Astrophobia (thunder and lightening)
- Claustrophobia (small spaces)
- Mysophobia (germs)
- Aerophobia (flying)
- Trypophobia (holes)

Other (interesting) phobias include:

Apiphobia	or the fear of	Bees
Bromidrophobia	or the fear of	Body smells
Cariophobia	or the fear of	Heart/Heart Diseases
Coprophobia	or the fear of	Feces
Dendrophobia	or the fear of	Trees
Dentalphobia	or the fear of	Dentists/ Dentistry
Emetophobia	or the fear of	Vomiting
Erythrophobia	or the fear of	Blushing/Color Red
Frigophobia	or the fear of	Cold/Cold Things
Gerontophobia	or the fear of	Elderly People/ Growing Old
Hippophobia	or the fear of	Horses

Ichthyophobia	or the fear of	Fish
Isolophobia	or the fear of	Being Alone
Kainophobia	or the fear of	New Things
Koniophobia	or the fear of	Dust
Ligyrophobia	or the fear of	Loud Noises
Lygophobia	or the fear of	Darkness
Mechanophobia	or the fear of	Mechanical Things
Molysmophobia	or the fear of	Being contaminated
Necrophobia	or the fear of	Dead Things/ Death
Ornithphobia	or the fear of	Birds
Social Phobia	or the fear of	Negative Evaluations in Social Settings
Technophobia	or the fear of	Technology
Zoophobia	or the fear of	Animals

A fear of one object or situation is called a **specific phobia**. Phobias which branch out, causing the same reaction for different or varied items are known as **complex phobias.** A fear of snakes that broadens to a fear of jump ropes or extension cords is an example of a complex phobia.

Although each individual's phobia battle is unique, hypnotherapy has the answer. The key to success, as I have regularly reported in these pages, is the client's very own mind – that is where the magic happens. The hypnotherapist plays an integral role in translating the issues to be addressed and goals being sought into language that the client's Middle Mind will process as the recipe for cooking up new, permanent behaviors in response to the phobias' triggers.

On a first visit, the hypnotherapist wants to accomplish several things. First, the therapist wants to get to know the client. Key information she will need includes how the client communicates and processes information. As the conversation narrows to the phobia, the hypnotherapist will explore the history of the phobia, using questions such as these:

- When did the phobia manifest and what were the circumstances?
- When did the phobia first begin to cause problems?
- What has been the worst phobic experience?
- Describe the last phobic experience.
- Are there others close to you who share similar phobias?
- Describe the specific details of this particular phobia. (What snakes bother you most? What height begins to cause you to panic? Does the size of the dog matter?)
- What benefits do you see from conquering this phobia?

Simply working through the background of your particular phobia may have some therapeutic benefit!

The therapist will next begin to explore the goals you want to achieve and the plan for in-session hypnotherapy. You will also work out your after-session application plans to practice the skills you are developing.

You will undergo hypnosis in order to investigate the problematic behavior and to supply your Middle Mind with the necessary language to reprogram your behavior. The goal is to desensitize you to the cause of your phobia. The objective is to develop a reasoned approach to the object or the situation that triggers your phobic behaviors. A myriad of technical approaches is available for the hypnotherapist to use, including developing an anxiety hierarchy, using regression therapy, or using neuro-linguistic programming. The options that hypnotherapy provides and the record of successes with treating phobias should provide any sufferer with the encouragement he or she needs to proceed with treatment!

CHAPTER 26

PTSD (POST-TRAUMATIC STRESS DISORDERS)

Hypnotherapy has proven valuable for treating the myriad of symptoms that can affect those suffering from Post-traumatic Stress Syndrome (PTSD). Once associated primarily with soldiers returning from war, this disorder is now recognized in conjunction with a variety of experiences. The origin of the problem begins with the experiencing or the witnessing of a traumatic event or events. Like a soldier in war or a child suffering from sexual abuse by an adult, the trauma may be a continuing series of events, lasting from days to years. The trauma may also come through all too common events that life brings, such as auto accidents, other serious injuries, or criminal attacks.

Some may experience a sense of recovery from any of these events, but a condition is labeled PTSD only if the symptoms last for more than a few months and begin to interfere with normal daily functions. Some of the typical symptoms include flashbacks of the traumatizing event(s), nightmares, anxiety (and all of its accompanying manifestations), and excessive thinking about the causative event(s).

Hypnotherapy can treat PTSD by working with the Middle Mind, the subconscious seat of the problem. A PTSD sufferer is continuously exposed to the traumatic events as the Middle Mind continuously re-plays those events, seemingly in an uncontrollable fashion. Therapy using hypnosis is critical to reaching those behaviors and altering them.

PTSD will intrude on other behavior and relationships, as well. This "cross contamination" takes place outside the conscious, rational mind, and once again, seems permanent, not subject to a willed, conscious change. Hypnotherapy offers techniques to get past these mental blocks in order to effectively rewire the brain's responses to the trauma.

As symptoms continue, clients with PTSD often seek relief that allows them to avoid the pain of the symptoms. This avoidance can take the form of addictive behavior as sufferers try to self-medicate to numb the pain. Many of those with PTSD turn to alcohol or drugs to avoid the pain. Others may turn to self-harm, and when the pain seems overwhelming, they may even attempt suicide. Increasing suicide rates nationwide are connected with PTSD who have lost hope in finding any relief.

The strain of dealing with the PTSD symptoms can result in physical and mental problems, in addition to the emotional ones. Many of these issues may simply be latent situations interfering little, if at all, with life. The stress and anxiety of the PTSD aggravate pre-existing conditions, adding to the sufferers' overall problems.

In hypnotherapy, treatment is tailored to the individual, specifically dealing with the person's personal manifestation of PTSD. The therapy will explore and dissociate the event(s) in order to reach a point in which the primary event may be addressed, but without the emotional responses and attendant symptoms. A sufferer may need to "let loose" those debilitating emotions in order to reach a type of closure or resolution. A therapist will help a sufferer to be de-sensitized to the situation. These clients will need ego-strengthening, the recall and reestablishment of their dominant strengths they inherently possess, as they work to restore themselves to a more normal functioning state. Hypnotherapy will also offer proven measures to help sufferers control behaviors that have led to addictive activities, self-harm, relationship issues, and health issues, both mental and physical.

With the incredibly broad range of symptoms of PTSD, hypnotherapy and its broad arsenal of behavior-changing weapons offers unique assistance for the suffering individual.

CHAPTER 27

EATING DISORDERS

A. Anorexia

Anorexia Nervosa is an emotional eating disorder which results in a two-pronged behavioral-emotional response. Behaviorally, a sufferer controls eating in order to lose weight. Emotionally, the behavior becomes a persistent and obsessive compulsion. Long-term anorexia has devastating consequences for a person's health, even leading to death. Since anorexia is a psychological disorder at its origin, hypnotherapy provides an effective and safe way to address the issues without the long-term costs of plodding psychotherapy or the unknown side-effects of psychotropic drugs.

Although the chief characteristics of anorexia are the same for most people, i.e., the obsessive desire to lose weight and the refusal to take in adequate nourishment, the causes and underlying emotional responses are unique to each person.

The unhealthy behaviors of anorexia clients have become

hard-wired over time into their Middle Minds (subconscious). [See CHAPTER 7] The harmful habits become hard-wired into the behavior because in its interpretation of the world around it, the mind misconstrues key information and attaches it to emotions. For example, critical comments about a child's weight might be the point of origin for the anorexia. Many adult behaviors are family influenced, and a family history of eating disorders might establish poor family habits and processing, as a whole. A person's work, social setting, or hobby may even supply the pressure and the attached emotions which make a person's body size obsession quite dangerous. Obsessive personalities in general, anxiety issues, relationship difficulties, and other stressors can all contribute to the emotional responses that mis-wire the Middle Mind's development of appropriate behavioral responses.

People with anorexia nervosa have a number of rather complex issues. One is that they do not have a true perception of their bodies. An anorexic sees herself as fat, even when she is dangerously thin and malnourished. She also sees food as the enemy, or at least an obstacle, that causes harm.

The complex combination of a distorted self-perception combined with an inherent but mis-applied need for approval will create a distorted overall self-image. Thus, the anorexic will feel inadequate in most situations, creating a sense of anxiety that grows daily.

Hypnotherapy provides the tools necessary to discover the root causes of the problem and to address the various components which create the health and emotional dangers. Therapists can help to introduce new behaviors that disrupt, remove, and replace the previous, unhealthy ones. As these new behaviors develop, the client will experience greater confidence and healthier self-esteem. With the therapist, the client will organize a nutritional intake management plan which will lead to more healthy eating practices. With these changes, the anxiety and daily stressors will come under more control, and the client's self-image will improve. The key to these changes will come through the amazing mind of the anorexic herself! The hypnotherapist will provide the means to supply the new data needed for change by safely using hypnosis. Utilizing this approach, the changes should come more rapidly than they would with other psychological approaches. Thus, costs should be lower, the risks that come with psychotropic drugs are avoided, and the results in behavior change will be permanent.

B. Bulimia and Binge Eating Disorder

Bulimia (Bulimia Nervosa) is a condition characterized by uncontrolled eating or binge eating, most often occurring in women (ninety percent of bulimics are women). During the binge, a bulimic eats enormous quantities of food, typically sweet, high calorie foods such as gallons of ice cream, whole loaves of bread, or entire cakes. The binge is likely the result of some trigger, a particular stress or anxiety that has formed as an ignition spark for the binging. During the binge, clients report that they often feel consciously absent from the eating. Almost always, the bulimic engages in his eating privately, and though she feels a loss of control during the binge, the control returns immediately if another person appears.

After binge eating, bulimics are overwhelmed with guilt.

Because they often have poor or punitive views of their bodies, their guilt drives them to take extreme and dangerous measures to prevent weight gain. Bulimics typically fall into one of two groups, depending on how they handle the guilt. Those who purge characteristically induce vomiting, but they also abuse laxatives and diuretics (using illegal drugs in some cases) or enemas to avoid weight gain. Those who do not purge resort to dangerous periods of physical exertion, such as extreme exercise or sudden and prolonged periods of fasting.

A psychological cousin of Bulimia Nervosa is simply known as Binge Eating Disorder. Those suffering from this disorder show most of the characteristics of bulimia, except for the extreme efforts to rid the body of the calories consumed during the binge. As a result, a person with Binge Eating Syndrome is inevitably obese.

One well-recognized profession associated with high cases of bulimia is the fashion modeling industry. We all recognize that in a profession which puts such strong demands upon body size for advancement, bulimia seems inevitable. However, bulimics need not be models. In fact, most of them are not. Many bulimics include our friends, our family, or our co-workers. Many suffer privately and would be horrified if their bulimia were discovered. The causes of the binge eating and the purging or calorie burning activities fueled by guilt spring from a number of different factors, crafted and solidified by emotions in the Middle Mind. [See CHAPTER 7].

Before starting hypnotherapy, which is particularly beneficial for bulimics, a hypnotherapist should insist that certain physical and medical issues be addressed by a medical professional. For instance, the stress from purging or other calorie burning efforts may cause dental problems, intestinal problems, and stomach issues. Drug use may result in dangerous body chemicals and addictions. The immediacy of these health risks means that they must be addressed before therapy. Only after a medical clearance should hypnotherapy commence.

Once therapy begins, using the client's personal history and the therapist's hypnosis, both the causes and the full psychological nature of the bulimia can be explored and identified. Together, the therapist and the client will use techniques that dislodge, breakdown, and otherwise disrupt the currently embedded behaviors. Once the control of these long-standing behaviors are weakened, the client will develop new methods of dealing with the emotional or psychological stressors. These new behaviors come via suggestions offered during hypnosis and are utilized by the client's own unique Middle Mind to form new healthy responses. Such responses will include higher levels of conscious activity and control to help create wise decisions and positive self-images. The client leaves the therapist ready to implement the changes and to make progress in the real world. Any challenges she may face can be addressed in subsequent sessions so that she and the therapist can develop steps to ensure that the new healthy behaviors are permanent improvements. Anyone suffering with bulimia should see a hypnotherapist as soon as possible. They need not suffer any more!

CHAPTER 28

DIGESTIVE AND GASTRO-INTESTINAL ISSUES

A. Irritable Bowel Syndrome (IBS).

Irritable Bowel Syndrome is an intestinal disorder causing some combination of abdominal pain, gas, bloating, diarrhea, and constipation. The diagnosis is usually made based upon the symptoms. In fact, lab tests and imaging are seldom employed in the medical analysis. The ailment is not curable, but some medical treatments can mitigate the severity of the symptoms, which can last for years or even for a lifetime. Most people first experience symptoms in their twenties. While some people may see reduced symptoms over time, others are just the opposite, experiencing worsening symptoms as they age. Certain foods, like those higher in fiber, or drinks, such as alcohol or caffeinated sodas, may trigger symptoms. While foods seem a likely culprit, (e.g., too much food or food that is fried or fatty) other triggers such as stress can also exacerbate the problem.

As IBS continues, some sufferers report a variety of other conditions. Some experience cramps, either in the bowels or in the rectum or both. Bowel movements fluctuate between diarrhea and constipation. Some sufferers have a feeling of urgency in urination that sends them running for bathrooms, an experience that can interfere with both social activities and work. Back pains that are related to alternating conditions of bowel movements, belching, and vomiting have also been connected with IBS.

Obviously, experiencing such symptoms impacts an individual psychologically. Embarrassment can create stress, which can lead to anxiety. As a result, sufferers tend to curtail their social activities, and life as a whole can begin to deteriorate. The condition consumes everything for the approximately 200,000 IBS sufferers in the United States.

But there is hope! Hypnotherapy has proven to be an effective means of managing the condition, eliminating or significantly lessening the symptoms, so that a client may return to a normal lifestyle.

We now know, and medical science agrees, that there is a brain-gut connection involved in such conditions. We also see that there are elements within the Middle Mind that either originate or exacerbate this condition [see CHAPTER 7], thus I like to refer to this connection as more of a Middle Mind – Gut Connection. Study after study shows the effectiveness of hypnosis-based therapy in improving a client's overall well-being, improving the quality of life, reducing or eliminating abdominal pain, and eliminating or reducing constipation, diarrhea, bloating, and gas. Fatigue, backache, and urinary problems have also shown improvement. At least seventy-five percent of those with IBS have benefitted significantly from hypnotherapy. Benefits of hypnotherapy are sustainable; therefore, clients will reach the cost benefit at the second year of therapy. Hypnotherapy, as one of its trademark benefits, is also faster in positive results than other types of counseling.

Hypnotherapy intervenes to stop the symptoms at several levels. It can give clients more instinctive control over their diets, similar to the control that it gives for weight loss clients. It can offer the same methodology for pain management as it does for those with chronic pain. Of course, hypnotherapy always proves quite effective in relaxing and managing stress, a most necessary task for those suffering from a condition as medically and emotionally confusing as IBS. IBS clients can also gain more confidence and brighter daily outlooks as they get this most aggravating condition under control.

B. Crohn's Disease and Ulcerative Colitis

Crohn's Disease is a chronic inflammation of the bowel that effects the lining of the digestive tract. It is a medically diagnosed disease that can last throughout a person's lifetime. Crohn's Disease causes abdominal pain, fever, bowel obstructions, blood in the stool, and diarrhea. Other symptoms from this disease include loss of appetite, nausea, aching joints, tiredness, and a plethora of other problems. Although there may be periods when a person is not experiencing symptoms, the other times of suffering can lead to such serious problems as bleeding, infection, kidney stones, eye ailments, and holes in the intestinal walls. Crohn's Disease itself is not deadly, but it can lead to more life-threatening conditions such as colon cancer. Once a doctor has medically diagnosed the disease through tests, the medical treatments can vary from the use of steroids to battle the inflammation to antibiotics that treat the inflections to nutritional supplements to counteract the lack of absorption in the intestines. Other medications may be prescribed to meet other symptoms, as well.

Ulcerative Colitis is very similar to Crohn's Disease. The only distinction, for the most part, involves the area of the intestinal wall that is affected. Crohn's affects the entire intestinal wall, while Ulcerative Colitis affects only the interior-most layer of the intestinal wall. For our purposes, we will address the two conditions as one.

Although both conditions last a lifetime, hypnotherapy has been medically proven to assist in placing symptoms in remission and keeping them there. As we have mentioned in the prior IBS section, the connection between the mind and the gut is well documented. As a matter of fact, hypnosis-based therapy is now part of most medical specialist trainings for gastroenterologists.

Hypnotherapy that addresses the various components of Crohn's Disease offers relief in many areas. Crohn's is not caused by stress, but stress can impact the symptoms associated with it. Since the symptoms themselves can induce stress, fighting with Crohn's is a never-ending compounding of those symptoms. Hypnotherapy offers sufferers the tools necessary not only to relax, but also to reduce the pain. Since diet impacts any gastrointestinal issue, diet management becomes critical during hypnotherapy.

To adequately deal with this disease, sufferers should consult with a certified medical hypnotherapist. Before consulting with a hypnotherapist, though, make sure to have a clear medical diagnosis of the disease. If you happen to be suffering with this incurable condition, get relief today.

CHAPTER 29

HAVING CHILDREN

A. Fertility

As many as one in seven couples report today that they are having trouble conceiving children. Couples spend billions of dollars annually in their attempts to overcome infertility. For those who do finally get pregnant, it is not unusual for them to have spent a year or more in their efforts. Many couples are waiting longer to start their families, and that wait can present obstacles, both physical and mental.

Once a physician has examined a couple and has identified and treated any physical barriers to conception, hypnotherapy can offer a fast, effective way of increasing success in conceiving. A familiar scenario, one that you may have heard and that I have witnessed in my own immediate family, illustrates why hypnotherapy is a perfect tool for struggling couples. I have a niece and a nephew born fewer than nine months apart. After struggling to have children for an extended period of time, my brother and his wife found out that they would be adopting a baby girl. Almost immediately thereafter, they became pregnant, and a baby brother arrived on the scene. It is a story repeated often for those who have adopted children.

The desire for children is a powerful, innate drive for most couples. Many women played with dolls throughout their childhoods, and the imagery and emotions of such play helped to develop the desire to have and mother babies. Many men develop their own desires for children, as well. If a family is put on hold, whether intentionally or not, a couple knows the "clock is ticking". With the passage of time, pressure to conceive naturally interferes with the relationship. Sometimes real physical obstacles to pregnancy may be the culprit to infertility. Not all physical issues will make pregnancy impossible, but they may warn the couple of the difficulty ahead, adding more pressure to the mix. In addition, the family dynamics of the couple themselves is affected by infertility. Neither spouse wants to disappoint the other, and there is real guilt on both sides during repeated failures to conceive. How do all of these pressures impact fertility, and how can hypnotherapy help?

These tensions manifest themselves into physical stress and emotional anxiety. [For more discussion regarding general anxiety and stress, see CHAPTER 21.] In regard to fertility, anxiety and stress bring about certain physical reactions that tend to hamper pregnancy. It is really very simple. When a person responds to life challenges, if severe enough, instinctive "fight or flight" type chemical reactions kick in. Chief among these reactions are hormonal changes, which tend to lower the chances of fertilization. With couples, there is double trouble as this hormonal challenge can hit both the male and female, inhibiting hormones that assist in fertilization in both partners. Since hypnotherapy is proven effective for stress and anxiety problems, it can serve as an effective tool for increasing fertility, either alone if no physical cause has been identified, or as a complement to support a couple that is also receiving medical and chemical assistance.

The hypnotherapist will get to know the couple or the individual seeking help in order to identify the conscious and unconscious challenges, review the couples' history, and to work with the client(s) to establish objectives and a plan to address the fertility challenge. The overall goal of therapy will be to enable the couple to relax enough that the mind and the body do not experience the intensity causing the physical reactions that obstruct fertility. Couples should be able to relax and enjoy the baby-making process, if you know what I mean.

Whether the issues include negative self-talk, wrong or unfair beliefs, guilt, or some other problematic behavior, hypnotherapy, utilizing hypnosis tactically, can give couples a relaxing, confident and enjoyable approach to a very exciting and fulfilling future.

B. Pain-Free Childbirth

The vast majority of women who have used hypnosis for one child inevitably use the method exclusively thereafter. What brings such great devotion to the wedding of hypnosis and childbirth?

The objective with hypnosis during childbirth is to allow the mother to experience a fully natural child birth, avoiding chemical and other medical pain management techniques typical of most deliveries today. Mothers often share their concerns with the side effects of these typical medical techniques, or their fears about procedures applied incorrectly, or their worries about extended recoveries. Today, many consider hypnosis-based childbirth to be the most effective method for natural childbirth.

Hypnotherapy provides a mother the techniques with which to deal with the fear, anxiety, and pain that most women experience during childbirth. Fear and anxiety bring emotional pressures that cause the body to become physically tense, slowing and exacerbating the entire process. Using hypnotic techniques, the mother remains calm, in control, mentally alert, and more able to fully participate in the miracle of childbirth.

God promised Eve that "in pain you shall bring forth children," and most women throughout history can confirm its severity. Hypnosis does not make the physical feeling of pain disappear. In fact, the total discomfort will not be gone at all, but those using hypnotherapy techniques report a new experience of the discomfort, a new understanding, a distinct re-focusing or re-packaging of the pain. A mother is able to refocus the pain, to push it to the background of thought, letting the mind concentrate on other ideas or experiences. Due to the more relaxed state of the mothers, the deliveries tend to advance faster, thus limiting her amount of time in pain.

Hypnotherapy is becoming more and more popular for expectant couples as they move toward more simple childbirth experiences. A mother and her partner can prepare with a hypnotherapist or with classes. On the date of delivery, the mother may have a therapist present, but more likely the couple will be schooled in techniques of self-hypnosis which generally proves successful for fully achieving the goals of a happy, drug-free, pain-controlled delivery.

C. Postpartum Depression (PPD)

Depression affects as many as fifteen percent of new mothers. An estimated eighty percent of mothers experience some elements of PPD after childbirth, and the symptoms are transitory. If the condition continues, mothers should seek help because PPD untreated can have sad consequences for mother, child, and the entire family.

[Note: Fathers can experience PPD as well, although a full-blown disorder occurs far more seldom than with mothers. For the purposes of this chapter, we will address only mothers, but a suffering father should definitely consider hypnotherapy for many of the same reasons discussed here.]

Postpartum depression presents a complicated combination of issues, but it is a disorder that hypnotherapy can untangle in order to assist the mother in managing and overcoming each symptom.

Once flippantly referred to as the "Baby Blues," PPD presents many serious and troubling symptoms. A PPD sufferer is likely to report many of the following conditions: mood swings, crying spells, irritability, anxiety, depression, self-doubting, visions or thoughts of harming self or child (including thoughts of suicide and murder), fits of rage, general lack of interest, sleeping problems (beyond the obvious ones associated with having a newborn in the house), eating problems (too much intake or too little), and difficulty bonding with the child. The condition can result in overwhelming guilt and embarrassment. If left untreated, beside the fact that the child is at risk of physical harm, the children from a mother with PPD can develop emotional and behavioral problems. A mother with severe PPD will often be confused, experience obsessive thoughts, delusions, and paranoia.

Researchers can point to no one culprit as the cause of PPD because of the complexity of all the changes occurring in the woman's body during pregnancy and childbirth. Mothers who already deal with mental or emotional issues, such as bipolar disorder, are at a higher risk for PPD. Even with no real history with these disorders, certain women with family histories of mental problems may also be predisposed to PPD. Physically, a woman's body after childbirth must heal from this traumatic event, and during this healing, significant hormonal changes occur. Added to the physical changes are the multiple life and family changes that can generally be characterized as "adjustments to motherhood." In one single event, all the family relationships and dynamics are altered. The mother may lack support, or at least sense a lack of support. Outside pressures that come with a job, finances, or social responsibilities may contribute to a rise in PPD. Just simple fatigue from being a new mom or a more serious health problem that mom and child may experience may add to the challenges. No wonder so many women are overwhelmed by PPD! It is a wonder that more of them are not!

Physicians tend to rely upon antidepressant drugs for

treatment of PPD. However, with the complexity of causes and symptoms we have just outlined, it is easy to see why drugs alone fall short of what a mother needs to overcome PPD. Talk Therapy, i.e. psychoanalytical styles of treatment with dozens of sessions over extended periods of time, may offer some relief. But many new mothers are already overwhelmed with time constraints and family obligations, and such an approach can be costly and time consuming.

Hypnosis-based therapy offers a faster, more flexible treatment plan. This book discusses many of the symptoms of PPD in earlier chapters, i.e., anxiety, stress, eating, sleeping. The hypnotherapist, as needed, can utilize the tools necessary in a treatment plan tailored to the mother's needs. In the first session, the therapist and the patient will work together to identify the immediate threat issues, develop the steps necessary to address them, and implement hypnosis to change them. Concern about physical injury is paramount, so a therapist must first work to neutralize any strong feelings about self-harm or harm to others. As they work through those immediate concerns, the therapist and the client will start to unpack the peripheral symptoms, working through not only the plethora of physical and social changes, but also the complex emotions that arise from pregnancy, childbirth, and recovery. The therapist will help the client work to re-program her confused Middle Mind, identifying the challenges, and developing a plan for recovery and restoration. In addition to dealing with each symptom, the mother will learn hypnosis-based techniques to handle the guilt and embarrassment she may experience, building more confidence and finally establishing a clear mental image of the joy of motherhood.

CHAPTER 30

CHILDREN AND ADOLESCENTS

T his section looks at pediatric problems and problems that may be affecting adults, but which originated in them as children or were identified in them during childhood. For our purposes here, the terms *child* or *children* will include those children through adolescence.

Hypnotherapy can be incredibly helpful in addressing many childhood problems, but there are major differences between their therapy and the therapy for adults. Let's look at some of the major distinctions.

1. Role of the parents. First, the parents play a key role in a child's therapy. In fact, the adults may have a greater motivation for change than the child. I prefer that the parent be present during the child's initial session, primarily because having them present is the most ethical option. Secondly, the parents' presence usually boosts confidence for both the parents and the child. Thirdly, the parent's feedback can prove helpful in evaluating the child's progress. However, there may be times where factors dictate that the hypnotherapist be alone with the child. As a child reaches those teenage years, he or she is more likely to view parents as a restriction to the sessions. Therapists will deal with such issues on a case-by-case basis.

2. Incentive to change. All therapy is initiated by a high level of desire for change. With adults, the decision to seek therapy in the first case is a highly personal one. A real measure of the incentive for an adult is monetary, the willingness to pay for therapeutic services. With a child, we lack the same signs of motivation. Children may even lack the adults' awareness that their behavior is anything outside of normal. What offsets this uncertainty in incentive is a child's natural inclination to follow the guidance of a parent combined with his or her developmental stage which actually makes hypnosis-based therapy in many ways easier and exceedingly transformational in children.

3. Children make outstanding hypnotic subjects. Oh, the imagination of children! They have the ability to create their own little worlds, the ability to transform into superheroes. I remember spending hours reinventing myself as my favorite baseball players, like Johnny Bench, or my favorite quarterbacks, like Broadway Joe Namath. Often, a child will have an imaginary friend. Some children will sneak books to be late at night because they are so enthralled with the stories. All of these acts demonstrate the incredible imagination of children. The natural willingness of children to enter into deep imaginative scenarios makes them excellent subjects for hypnosis. They do not question "Why?" at every step, and their developing forms of reasoning are open to anything new. As they play, children are already experiencing a form of self-hypnosis, and play is essential in a child's Middle Mind development. Harnessing this playing-learning capability makes hypnotherapy for children extraordinarily effective.

Not only is hypnosis almost a game for the child (and sometimes for the therapist, too!), it also allows the child to go deeper into a productive trance stage faster. While in this stage, a child is extraordinarily suggestible, willing to accept and capture ideas offered by the therapist. As a result, children often experience faster results.

Let's now look at some of the more common issues associated with children. We will follow that with problems which may affect adults as well as children, but whose characteristics have probably impacted the adults since childhood.

A. Anxiety

Anxiety in children is almost too broad a category to address here. However, we will discuss some symptomatic behavior, such as bedwetting, in this section. Children and adolescents, however, face their own versions of practically every issue that we have already discussed in this text. Obesity in children continues to grow. Eating disorders are also prevalent and growing among the young. Children also develop stutters or develop other speech problems in conjunction with anxiety. School itself presents a number of pressures that produce anxiety, from public speaking to test-taking. The interactions with parents, teachers, and peers trigger many emotional and psychological challenges. Studies now show that graduating high school students are entering the world with self-esteem levels at the lowest levels ever measured. Depression and high suicide rates are an ever-increasing source of concern. Technology has retarded social skill development. Vaping (CHAPTER 23), Video games (CHAPTER 35), and Pornography (CHAPTER 31) have created unique manifestations of anxiety among teenagers. What the future holds for our youth under such social pressures defies our imagination.

Some of the problems that children face are uniquely developmental problems, but chief among those developmental problems is anxiety, which so often lies at the heart of all other problems. Anxiety and its resolution both lie within a child's Middle Mind (CHAPTER 7). Blessedly, even when the children are teenagers, Middle Minds are more malleable; thus, hypnotherapy can reach more quickly the child's mind which governs behaviors and provides the raw ingredients to reprogram instincts, habits, and drives.

The fascinating power and complexity of the mind is just now beginning to be understood in terms of its strength and flexibility. But, through hypnotism, we have now discovered and learned to utilize this power in order to facilitate change. For children, the steps in hypnotherapy follow a basic pattern:

1. The therapist with the parents and the child determine the issue(s) to be addressed.
2. The therapist will ensure a comfortable setting to help discover the child's interests and level of communication. This information will guide the sessions, particularly the hypnotic suggestions.

3. The hypnotherapist will design suggestions for the child to utilize in forming new behaviors.
4. With a plan unique to the child based upon his or her age, communication skills, and interests, the child will be hypnotized and given the mental material needed to convert old behaviors into new ones.
5. The therapist will evaluate progress, using the evaluations to develop and implement post-session steps and follow-up.
6. The therapy is concluded when permanent behavior change occurs, something that often can be done rapidly with hypnotherapy.

With this process in mind, let us look briefly at several children's issues.

B. Bedwetting (Enuresis)

One common childhood problem that hypnotherapy can treat is bedwetting. Although it is considered a childhood problem, some adults battle it, as well. It occurs a bit more frequently in children of parents who themselves were bedwetters.

Generally, bedwetting is not a concern during the first three years of life, as children naturally have accidents as they transition out of diapers and develop bladder control. Some slower developing children take longer to control this problem though. Typically, therapy is not sought until a child is six years old or older.

Boys are more commonly nocturnal bedwetters (nocturnal enuresis), which is the most common form of bedwetting.

Daytime wetting (diurnal enuresis) is more common in girls.

Wetting the bed is a developmental issue that can develop from physical or mental causes. In most circumstances, a hypnotherapist will require that any physical/medical cause of the problem be address prior to entering into therapy. If no physical cause of the bedwetting is diagnosed, then the likely cause is psychological, and psychological causes are readily treated with hypnotherapy.

Bedwetting is one of those conditions which compounds problems. Such children often face the expressed displeasure of parents and are teased by their siblings. Any mention of the condition with other children brings shame and embarrassment. Social engagements, such as sleep-overs and camping trips, are avoided. With each embarrassment comes more pressure and anxiety. Conscious efforts by the child often backfire since the rule of reverse consequences takes over: as the child concentrates on avoiding the behavior, he actually reinforces it. The poor child is left frustrated, embarrassed, and hopeless. Long-term effects of bedwetting will undoubtedly lead to low self-esteem and other developmental problems.

Using hypnosis-based therapy, a therapist can addressed the Middle Mind (the subconscious; see CHAPTER 7) of the child where the bedwetting behavior originates. Hypnotherapy can address many behaviors tied to problems directly, so that bedwetters will be given suggestions to limit beverages before bedtime, to automatically wake-up before needing to urinate, and to exercise better control of the bladder. The overall mental picture a therapist will work to develop subconsciously in the child's mind is the experience of waking to a dry bed, and the joy and confidence from that experience. A child's mind is incredibly flexible enough to adjust behaviors, and hypnotherapy is an incredibly flexible tool that can bring rapid results.

C. Nightmares

Nightmares are not real, factual events, so where do they come from? Obviously, the answer lies in the mind, or more specifically, the Middle Mind (CHAPTER 7). For a developing mind like that of a child's, all sorts of mis-programming can corrupt the action within the Middle Mind. Hypnotherapy offers help to children who have persistent and frightening nightmares.

Through discussions before and during the hypnosis sessions, a therapist can identify the psychological causes of the nightmares. Once these causes are identified, the therapist can present subconscious directions to the child through the Middle Mind that will provide the tools the child needs not only to avoid the triggers of the nightmares, but also to cope with any peripheral nightmare issues.

Additional details on sleep disorders are presented in CHAPTER 22, and those discussions are relevant with children, as well.

D. Nail-biting

"Stop biting your nails!" For many of us, hearing that command repeatedly was enough. For others, however, biting our nails became a habit that has lasted far longer than it should.

My wife discovered a sure-fire method for her nail-biting habit. She bit her nails into her early twenties, but with the birth of her first child, she decided to use cloth diapers. After rinsing these diapers in the bathroom toilet, the act of bringing her hands to her mouth to bite her nails suddenly became a conscious act, one that was she quickly gained control over. Her habit had been a childhood one that followed her into adulthood. Because of its early onset, I include this problem with childhood problems, even though many adults still struggle with it. I will never forget meeting an attractive lady whose hands were a mess from her nail-biting habit. That's unfortunate because hypnotherapy provides a ready and quick answer to the problem.

Hypnosis-based therapy provides the perfect expedited method to stop biting fingernails. A long exploration of the cause or origin of the problem is not necessary here. It is clear what is happening: the nail biting occurs automatically, or as those in psychology might say, unconsciously. We hypnotherapists point to the subconscious as the point of origin, or as I would say, the Middle Mind (CHAPTER 7). What we are describing is simply an "unthinking" habit or instinct. Such behavior happens without any forethought. After the damage is done, the frustration and embarrassment begins. But something seems to be blocking the sufferer from getting control over the problem. And here lies the crux of the matter. Nail biting is an out-of-control behavior, but it is not a hopeless behavior. The secret to changing the behavior is to gain control of it; getting control begins with gaining awareness.

The automatic behavior of nail biting begins in the Middle Mind. It is an action that takes place in a non-thinking phase.

Hypnosis allows the client, with the assistance of the therapist, to first reach the point of origin in the Middle Mind. The previous automatic action can then be moved from the subconscious Middle Mind to the conscious-thinking mind. The goal, and the successful exercise of control, occurs when the client becomes consciously aware of the practice before it happens. After therapy, the client will become aware of his or her hand moving toward the mouth. For many people, this act seems quite simple, but for the nail-biter struggling with the problem, this awareness is a significant first step.

Once a client develops this awareness, he or she can then implement techniques to redirect or stop the nail biting altogether. Now the client has the control to stop the troublesome habit. It is time to invest in a good pair of nail clippers and set an appointment for a manicure!

For the nail biter, a few sessions of hypnotherapy results in a lifetime of control. This control will lead to a happier, confident life, day by day.

E. Thumbsucking

A common activity for young children, thumbsucking can ultimately lead to trouble and embarrassment for those who continue the habit into adulthood. The origins of thumbsucking, for therapeutic reasons, need not be explored, since it is so common for babies and toddlers. Only when the behavior does not naturally end should intervention be considered. If parents have been unsuccessful in breaking the habit in a child who is verbal and communicative, then they should seek help before problems set in.

Delaying intervention could lead to a host of problems as a child matures. One primary problem occurs in a child's dental health. For those who continue to suck their thumbs, the mouth and teeth begin to form around the thumb, creating dental malformations. These malformations, in turn, will lead to speech impediments. Children's health can be compromised due to a higher risk of illnesses from viruses, bacteria, and infections. For children, harassment and embarrassment from peers can create additional social pressures. For adults who continue to suck their thumbs, the problems are amplified.

Thumbsucking is an unconscious behavior (actually, more of a subconscious Middle Mind behavior; see CHAPTER 7). It is not a rational behavior that children decide to adopt, so some non-thinking benefit is obviously enjoyed by the thumbsucker. It may be a soothing or comforting gesture. It may be a mechanism developed in order to deal with stressors. For some, it may be a sleep aid. Ironically, those who suck their thumbs do so frequently in order to achieve a light, trance-like state, and, as a result, they are often excellent candidates for hypnosis-based therapy.

Results utilizing hypnotherapy may be achieved rather quickly. During the therapy, the goal consists of at least a three-fold objective. With techniques unique to hypnotherapy, the therapist will reach areas of the Middle Mind the client has not accessed, re-programming it so that the client will have a conscious awareness of the habit. Thus, the unconscious habit becomes a conscious one. The second objective is to create an aversion to the habit. Thirdly, the therapist will give suggestions that positively reinforce the benefits of living without the thumbsucking behavior. On top of the basic objectives, the therapist will work with the Middle Mind to bolster a client's overall confidence, self-esteem, and positive outlook on a non-thumbsucking life.

The brief time and minimal investment necessary to retrain the Middle Mind makes hypnotherapy a wise choice in treatment, for both children and adults.

F. Habit Cough

Habit Cough, or psychogenic cough or cough tic, is a rather unknown condition for most of us. It affects children and adolescents, but rarely affects adults. It can persist for years without intervention. Hypnotherapy has proven successful in the treatment of habit cough ninety percent of the time within a few session.

The continuing condition has no identifiable physical cause. The onset is often connected with a cold, the flu, or a respiratory infection. Sometimes, clients have asthma which may be a contributor to the condition. In very rare cases, the cough may originate with exercise or eating.

Studies reveal an interesting circumstance that is most revealing as to the psychological nature of the condition. Sometimes the actual physical illness associated with the beginning of the cough occurs when the child is experiencing emotional stressors. For example, some children develop the cough when a parent suffers from a serious illness, marital problems, serious mental conditions, or death.

The cough is often loud and harsh, occurring as often as several times a minute. Interestingly, it only happens when children are awake, not while they sleep, which also points to the automatic, subconscious, psychological nature of the condition. Something in the Middle Mind programming is instinctively, uncontrollably, triggering the urge to cough.

The persistent cough can lead to physical irritation and fatigue. The continuation of the cough can not only cause a child embarrassment, but it can also interfere with classroom work and other childhood activities. Of course, anxiety sets in if the cough is particularly interfering, which serves only to reinforce the habit. Cough suppressants and other medications are totally ineffective in treating the condition.

The hypnotherapist will seek to comfort the child and create confidence for the child in the hypnosis-based therapy. The goal is to use the Middle Mind's amazing abilities to reset itself. Using suggestions as the raw material of recovery, the hypnotherapist will provide the child with avoidance/distraction tools to suppress the cough. These tools will combine with additional processes that allow the child to retain conscious control of the behavior. In time, the new, improved non-coughing behavior will simply become second nature to the child, and the coughing issue will end.

Hypnosis-based therapy is a proven fast, safe, and highly recommended treatment option for children and their parents. Do not delay if this habit is affecting your family!

G. Attention Deficit Disorder (ADD) and Attention Deficit Hyperactivity Disorder (ADHD)

As with so many of the childhood problems we have already discussed, ADD or ADHD symptoms often appear early but continue into adulthood. For the purposes of this section, our references to ADD will include the sub-type ADHD, as well as the less common sub-type Attention Deficit Inattentive Disorder, a form characterized by "spacing out" or daydreaming.

ADD is not a problem that can be cured. Thus, the goal of all treatment is to control the symptoms. As a result, hypnotherapy is a most successful tool in the battle. We will first look at the causes of the symptoms, the nature of the symptoms, and the effects not only on children, but also on adults. We will follow that with a review of treatments and, ultimately, the goals of hypnotherapy for children or adults with ADD.

The problems with ADD originates in the brain. Brain scans show that the cortex of the brain, where thinking takes place, is asleep in those with ADD symptoms. More specifically, the pre-cortex, the very front of the cortex, is not functioning. This part of the brain filters all the stimuli that a person encounters. For those with ADD, the brain is simply overwhelmed. [For those who have read the explanations about the Middle Mind in CHAPTER 6 and CHAPTER 7, you can immediately see why hypnotherapy may be a serious option for treating ADD. Consider, if the thinking, conscious mind is asleep, what part of the brain is calling the shots? The only reasonable conclusion is that the subconscious or Middle Mind is in charge. Since hypnosis is key to accessing the Middle Mind, it is clear how important hypnotherapy can be in the treatment of ADD.] ADD is more common in males and is typically diagnosed when a child begins school.

What causes the differences of the brains of those with ADD? It may be heredity, or it may be an innate genetic issue. Brain diseases or injuries may contribute to it. Activities of the mother during pregnancy, such as drinking alcohol, using drugs, or smoking, may be a factor. Toxins or other chemical exposures may be catalysts, as well. Finding a simple cause such as a chemical imbalance or determining the exact nature of the onset of ADD is actually a rare occurrence, so finding a cure for these symptoms may be impossible.

All of the symptoms of ADD are behavioral, once again pointing to the value of hypnotherapy as a highly effective treatment. Characteristics of ADD include short attention span, forgetfulness, distractibility, impulsiveness, procrastination, disorganization, poor planning, and failure to complete tasks. ADHD adds the additional symptom of hyperactivity and is probably by far the most commonly diagnosed.

For children, ADD impacts almost every aspect of their lives. They experience problems with nearly all learning activities related to school work. They have trouble reading books or focusing on anything that requires concentration. Many times, discipline issues arise, and in later years these issues can grow into criminal behaviors. Of course, with all these problems, children face stunted social development, poor relationships with peers or family, and low self-esteem. Ultimately depression and anxiety can overwhelm them.

In adults, ADD manifest itself in a variety of ways. Those with ADD are often chronically late and suffer with low self-esteem and anxiety. Some struggle to manage their frustrations and anger, while others turn to alcohol or drugs to cope.

The most common form of medical treatment is the use of

pharmaceuticals, primarily stimulants. Obviously, the goal of the physician is to activate the part of the brain that is typically asleep, particularly that part of the brain which is failing to filter the overwhelming stimuli. Since some of these drugs work really well at activating the brain, the behaviors can change dramatically and quickly. A single dose can completely change a client's demeanor, behavior, and even his handwriting.

In a world interested in organic foods and all natural products, the problems with the standard medical treatments are obvious. With these chemicals, what are the long-term consequences? Short term side effect for stimulant-based medication includes nervousness and irritability, sleep problems, decreased appetite and weight loss, increased blood pressure, dizziness, moodiness, headaches, and stomach aches. Less common side effects include increased behavioral tics and personality changes. Non-stimulant medication actually causes many of the same side effects with the addition of fatigue, drowsiness, and mood swings.

Hypnotherapy offers either an alternative or a complementary tool to medication. Since hypnotherapy is all about changing behaviors, and since ADD treatment is all about controlling behaviors, applying hypnosis-based techniques to ADD symptoms proves quite successful.

The objective of therapy is to use hypnosis to empower the client and the Middle Mind to make the changes. The first goal is to relax and quiet the mind so that the behaviors can be modified. The client needs to be able to focus, concentrate, retain, and recall. Young clients will develop the skills needed to control behaviors such as fidgeting and impulsiveness.

They will learn to adjust behaviors in social situations and in educational settings. Older more mature clients may work to address planning, procrastination, and follow-through behaviors.

The length of the therapy will vary depending upon the number and seriousness of behavioral problems, but we are not talking about years of treatment like that found in psychotherapy. Hypnotherapists pride themselves on the speed in which clients can change their behaviors. For the person or family impacted by ADD, hypnotherapy offers safe and rapid results.

H. Tourette's Syndrome

The onset of Tourette's Syndrome typically occurs between the ages of two and fifteen, with the average onset around six years old. It affects boys three to four times more than girls, and it can last a lifetime, although symptoms typically lessen during adulthood. Hypnotherapy, either as an alternative to or as a complement with chemically-based treatments, has become well recognized as an effective and rapid way to help Tourette's sufferers deal with their symptoms.

Tourette's Syndrome is characterized by repetitive movements, repetitive sounds, or a combination of both. These tics happen intermittently throughout the day, even occurring during sleep. The condition can be mild or severe, simple or complex. Simple cases involve a single movement or sound, whereas a complex disorder involves more than one muscle group. The exact cause of Tourette's is unknown, but there is speculation that it has a genetic component as well as an environmental factor. Diagnosis of Tourette's is made strictly by observations and the reported family history.

The repetitive movements come in a wide variety of forms, from eye blinking, to head jerking, to shoulder shrugging, to mouth movements, and beyond. For those who make repetitive sounds, the variety of sounds is extensive: coughing, grunting, throat cleaning, barking, repeating phrases, repeating words that others speak, cursing obscenities.

Often Tourette's does not appear in a child as a lone condition. It has been associated with ADHD (see Section G above), Obsessive Compulsive Disorder, sleep disorders (see CHAPTER 22 and Section C above on nightmares), depression (see CHAPTER 38), anxiety (see CHAPTER 21), related physical pain and headaches (CHAPTER 19), and anger management issues (see CHAPTER 37). Because of the proven success of hypnosis-based therapy with these associated conditions, it is easy to see why hypnotherapy would be successful with Tourette's Syndrome.

Medical doctors will try to control the symptoms of Tourette's using a wide variety of drugs. They may try ADHD stimulants, antidepressants, epilepsy seizure medications, and many others. However, there is no single medical approach that seems to have gained prominence in treating the symptoms of this disorder.

During hypnotherapy, the therapist will address the symptoms by having the child learn to relax. Using suggestions during hypnosis, the child's Middle Mind or subconscious (see CHAPTER 7) is provided the information it needs to automatically (a) identify when a behavioral tic is imminent, (b) suppress or control the movement, and (c) finally to stop the behavior altogether. Ultimately, the child will recognize the triggers leading to the behavior, whether external or subconscious, and will be able to avoid them instinctively. Sometimes, the child/client will be given an alternative, much more subtle, action to replace the more obvious and distracting tic.

Additionally, the hypnotherapist will work with the client to rebuild confidence and self-belief. The therapist will also address those associated conditions, such as anxiety or ADHD or any of the others listed above. Depending upon the age of the child, some elementary training in self-hypnosis may be included in order to strengthen the results.

Generally, parents are surprised by how quickly a child can experience results with hypnotherapy. Sometimes the goals are reached within one or two sessions per tic. The therapist, however, will evaluate the exact nature of the tic(s) and the associated challenges in order to determine a solid outline of services. Blessedly, though, the future for children with Tourette's can be more hopeful through the use of hypnotherapy.

CHAPTER 31

PORNOGRAPHY

Amerca, we have a pornography problem. If you or a loved one is addicted to pornography, you are not alone. Hypnotherapy may offer you the freedom you need from this most devastating addiction.

Pornography, in one form or another, has always plagued mankind. While the advent of the printing press and the rise in magazines may have led to a spike in the usage of and the problems associated with porn, those cannot compare to the impact that we have experienced with the onset of the digital age. Pornography is simply a few clicks away, practically anywhere at any time.

Thirty percent of all data transferred across the Internet is porn-related. Pornography is a $12 billion dollar industry in the United State, and $97 billion worldwide. Sites dedicated to pornography are visited more often than Netflix, Amazon, and Twitter combined.

Individually, the statistics are overwhelming. Sixty-four percent of all young people ages 13-24 seek out porn at least weekly. By college, 90% of both college males and females are using porn. Just under 50% of males of all age groups and just under 20% of all women use porn weekly.

The usage of pornography affects not only individuals, but also families and communities as a whole. Studies show that men and women who view porn regularly are most likely to be verbally and physically aggressive. Girls between the ages of 14 – 19 who view pornography are more likely to be sexually harassed or assaulted. Divorce rates are twice as high in marriages where one spouse is a porn user, and that number is even greater among young couples. It is estimated that over half of all divorces are directly impacted by pornography.

So, when does viewing pornography become addicting? At what point should a person consider therapy? When a person feels the need to view porn in order to get through the day, or when he or she feels helpless to stop or that the habit is out of control, help is needed. Like drug addicts, a porn viewer may feel the need for more or stronger pornography. Many addicts spend as many as ten hours a day or more viewing porn. While there may be physical signs that accompany porn use, the most serious problems are the ones that impact relationships, family, and employment. With any of these issues, people must seek the help that they need.

Pornography is particularly devastating because of the spiral of destruction that it creates. The fantasy it creates may lead to an increased dissatisfaction with existing relationships, which in turn leads to increased porn use, which leads to increased dissatisfaction in the relationships. The barrier porn creates in the relationship tends to lead to loneliness, which leads to increased porn use. The pattern continues, and the user never really finds a sense of fulfillment.

Once a person can admit that, at least to some extent, he has lost control, he is admitting that "Something in me is running my life that I can't control 'consciously'." Thus, the Middle Mind, beyond the typical reach of the conscious mind, is in play with this addiction (see CHAPTER 7). As we have already discussed, hypnosis is the best tool to use to reprogram that Middle Mind so that an addict may change his behavior.

In hypnotherapy, we deconstruct the pornography addiction. The therapy allows the client to relax, letting his world that seems so out of control begin to slow down. He moves toward reestablishing control over his life and to consciously alter his behavior. He will repeatedly strengthen that control in therapy, building greater confidence as he progresses.

Undoubtedly, the addiction to pornography will have generated damage, misconceptions, and practical consequences that the client will need to address. Whether the addiction is a totally private matter or whether it has drawn the attention of family members or colleagues, the client may face guilt, humiliation, or embarrassment. Beyond that, recovering from porn addiction means healing broken or bruised relationships, not just remedying prior damage, but also establishing healthier views of what a real, loving relationship means.

As a part of healing those relationships, clients in general need to change their views from using people as objects for self-gratification to seeing individuals as having value, deserving respect, worthy of admiration, and needing nurturing. Ultimately, as people go through therapy, they will learn to rearrange their worlds to some degree, restoring balance, increasing productivity, and managing time more efficiently.

As ugly as pornography addiction is, hypnotherapy offers the tools necessary to clean it up and to free a soul.

CHAPTER 32

GAMBLING

T hey were part-time antique dealers in north Florida. I happened to be visiting their home on other business, but we began to talk about their antiques. A person could not move around in the house, it was so crammed full of furniture. The small warehouse out back looked the same. They apologized for the appearance and told this story. Business was good and bad. Antiques had flooded the market at ridiculously low prices. They were much cheaper to dealers, but the resale market was seriously depressed. The result was an overabundance of inventory. I asked about the cause and received an inside look at what gambling can do, not just to individuals, but also to an entire culture.

Casino gambling had recently been legalized in Mississippi, and casinos opened all along the state's Gulf coast. Heirlooms that filled the homes of families for generations in Mississippi, Alabama, and Louisiana were sold off at fire sale prices to fuel newly discovered gambling habits. These casinos darkened lives, shattering families, as sleepy, warm nights visiting on the front porches were now replaced with bright, flickering lights and unrealistic hopes. Family treasures, the antiques, were gone, but so much more had been lost. The individual and societal costs of gambling had ventured south. Another war was lost. For many, another period of reconstruction lay ahead.

Gambling provides an emotional rush. For some, it is an addiction as strong as any drug. It can be found not only at the casinos, but also online, or with a bookie, or by simply stopping by the Quick Mart for a scratch off or two on the way home from work. While many gamblers are adults who are lured into the temptations later, others begin as early as young adults in high school or college.

Everyone knows the odds. Everyone knows "the House" always wins. When one state began debating the feasibility of a state lottery, I saw a bumper sticker that stuck with me: "The Lottery – a tax on people that are bad at math." And yet we still gamble. Why?

Even for a single recreational player, gambling provides the thrill of the moment, the chemical rush throughout the body, which keeps a gambler coming back to the tables. Sure, the hope of riches is what initially captures and then continuously fuels the behavior. The desire to escape the current reality will always motivate some people, but at "that moment," it is that shot of hopeful adrenaline that drives those people back. Individuals become addicts when they lose all control. They act not out of pleasure alone, but out of compulsion, out of a need for a fix. Matters of finance, of family, or of job no longer take priority. An overwhelming instinct, originating deep within the person (which we know as the Middle Mind, or subconscious) is fully in control. The gambler may carry on a sensible debate with himself in the conscious mind, but he loses every time.

Hypnotherapy is key to stopping a gambling addiction. That compulsion cannot be controlled by willpower, discipline, rational thinking, or logical debate. Despite the time-consuming hours spent in talk therapy – counseling that can go on for months and years – trying to "think away" the habit, ultimately many will return to the habit.

Gambling is a subconscious habit. Of course, a gambler knows consciously what he is doing. However, as with all habits, he is simply observing his behavior rather than controlling his behavior. It is as if an animalistic instinct is driving him; and it is.

All habits originate in the Middle Mind (see CHAPTER 7). In the Middle Mind, all life experiences are warehoused, and the controls of many driving functions operate. We do not have to consciously think in order to walk; we just do it. Our hearts do not have to be told to beat; they just do it. These are necessary human functions operating in the subconscious. A problem occurs, however, when a harmful habit, like gambling, takes on the unconscious characteristics of an automatic function.

Hypnosis provides the only tool possible to reach into the Middle Mind effectively. It is the "bridge to the subconscious." Hypnosis does not solve the problem in and of itself; it provides access to the client to reach into his or her own subconscious Middle Mind, and then, with the direction and assistance of a therapist, to alter behavior permanently. Once hypnosis provides the access into the Middle Mind, the hypnotic suggestions become the tools with which behavior can be changed. These precisely worded phrases and sentences become the natural ingredients that the client's mind will use to make changes.

The main goal of hypnosis is to take the unconscious gambling habit and push it into the rational-thinking consciousness where odds and finances and family and work and other relevant factors will be logically analyzed so that a gambler can begin to make wise decisions. The gambler will use the Middle Mind to create new, calm control over the process. With hypnosis, gamblers will implement the suggestions to create aversions to the risks of gambling and to develop positive thoughts of a life under control, thus pushing out the false highs of the gambling rush. Now conscious will power and discipline will appear automatically, working for the client's well-being.

Hypnotherapy is the only process that offers the opportunity to rapidly change behavior this way, a way that produces permanent change, free from destructive habits.

CHAPTER 33

ALCOHOLISM

We know that hypnotherapy works well for overcoming addiction to alcohol because of the proven track record and credibility of Alcoholics Anonymous (AA). Let me explain. At its heart, AA is an ongoing, long term behavior control program. The meetings are actually forms of group therapy, a type of talk therapy. Because such talk therapy methods do not effect permanent changes, AA regularly applies a group discipline through the repetitiveness and peer pressure of group meetings. AA understands the control that alcohol has on behavior and the difficulty in restraining that behavior. Long term programs buttress an individual's will power and discipline, but these conscious efforts cannot reach and permanently correct a behavior like drinking. Hypnotherapy, however, can.

The element that distinguishes hypnotherapy from all other treatments for alcoholism is hypnosis. Some people can safely control their consumption of alcohol, monitoring the types and amounts of the alcohol they consume, avoiding any short term or long term issues. Others, regrettably, simply lose control on a daily basis or on binge drinking occasions. Many, feeling hopeless, may assign blame to a genetic predisposition, or to an alcoholic parent, or some other cause. However, the bottom line is that alcoholics have a dangerous habit, one that can control their actions, even when they consciously desire something altogether different. Whatever the origin of the behavior, we now understand that the powerful behavior is programmed into the individual's mind – the Middle Mind (see CHAPTER 7). Only hypnotherapy provides access to that programming, and that is done with hypnosis, the bridge to the subconscious.

Hypnosis allows a person to bypass the conscious mind, the thinking mind of will power and discipline that has failed the alcoholic, allowing the drinker in conjunction with a therapist to address and renovate the behavioral structure. Hypnosis is a super-relaxed condition which is highly focused, unlike sleep. All outside clutter is shut out so that an individual's mind may receive new programming which comes in through the language of the therapist. The client's own mind will then take these suggestions and, in due course, re-write the aberrant behavior. Once the behavior is changed at this level, the objective is for the change to be permanent and life-long.

The nature of alcoholism requires two major issues to be addressed: the chemical dependency and the habit. The drinker is physically addicted to the alcohol. The body craves it, demands it. Withdrawal produces a variety of challenging physical responses. Navigating these withdrawal symptoms often proves to be too challenging for an individual alone, and an effort to become sober fails at the first effort. With hypnosis, the client can be empowered to relax and provide the Middle Mind with programming that successfully maneuvers through the physical challenges. The pain and discomfort associated with withdrawal can be compartmentalized and reduced with hypnosis. An alcoholic will have the confidence and the positive attitudes necessary to weather the process during hypnotherapy.

In addition to the chemical dependency is the habit itself. I would describe the habit as more powerful than simply being part of the drinker's lifestyle, although that is certainly a part of it. Times and events serve as triggers to the alcoholic's behaviors. To subconsciously change behaviors, the Middle Mind requires programming that instinctively defeats the triggers, providing an automatic and positive response to those triggers.

Through both parts of hypnotherapy, a therapist will employ very practical strategies. From the initial session, the hypnotherapist in concert with the client will develop a game plan for winning the battle. Hypnosis will be the tool to pinpoint the heart of the behavioral change, but real world application is the real test. The client is not simply turned out in the cold world alone to struggle with the challenges. The plan will create opportunities for proactive reporting on follow-up sessions, fine-tuning behaviors and strategies as the client faces real world experiences. Both the client and the therapist want success, and together they will find the answers.

A person seeking hypnotherapy for alcohol abuse is generally sufficiently motivated to change, a key to any successful hypnotherapy process. With the client's desire as a solid starting point, the exciting future of a life under control lies ahead. Hypnotherapy works.

CHAPTER 34

DRUG ADDICTION & SUBSTANCE ABUSE

D rug addiction grows as a serious problem each year. In my home community, the opioid crisis has taken many young lives. As a result of cultural changes, we are seeing more disillusioned young people who do not know how to face the world in which they live. They are more prone to seek escape by experimenting with drugs. For those caught up in substance abuse and addiction, hypnotherapy is effective in guiding them toward recovery and clean living.

The addiction to drugs is first and foremost a chemical addiction. A hypnotherapist will typically not begin sessions with a client until the physical addiction has been addressed and controlled. Confronting aberrant behaviors works most effectively when the client is clear-headed, communicative, and committed to change. Managing the physical condition sets the stage for progress and hypnotherapy.

Studies show that treatment utilizing hypnosis is more effective than talk therapy treatment for substance abuse.

Why is this the case? Hypnotherapy allows for the change in the cause of behavior. Behaviors originate in the Middle Mind (see CHAPTER 7), which is to say that the driving forces behind behaviors are not conscious thoughts. In fact, most substance abusers avoid thoughts which show the destruction and mayhem from the addiction. Try as they may to change, they continue to act in a way they do not want to act. They know the physical cost, the financial cost, the cost to family, and the destruction of their futures, and yet they still pursue the next fix. This drive, this instinct, this habit, all originate within drug user, but it does not seem to be controlled by the drug user. There exist behaviors and emotions that contribute to beginning the substance abuse in the first place, and there exist behaviors and emotions enabling the continued abuse.

Behavior cannot be changed by education. Behaviors cannot be changed by repetition. Behaviors reside in the Middle Mind and the Middle Mind can be accessed in only one way, through hypnosis. Hypnosis is the gateway to the subconscious. It is in the subconscious, the Middle Mind, where behaviors are locked in. While hypnosis, in and of itself, will not change behavior, it is the tool that allows the therapist to access the programming of the client's behavior. Knowing how and when to use hypnosis, as well as how to employ other tools in conjunction with hypnosis to bring about changes, is the job of the hypnotherapist.

Behaviors are originally created by a combination of factual circumstances wedded to emotional experiences. Many of the behaviors that we have as adults are formed in childhood. As children, behaviors are ill-formed by misunderstandings, misinterpretations, and traumatic events. Once formed, these behaviors become locked in, many times becoming irreversible.

Two types of behaviors affect substance abusers. There are general behaviors that have wide-ranging impact on the individual's entire life. These might be behaviors that generate anxieties, stresses, and other conditions that could set the stage for developing a drug habit. Then when the drug habit begins, the chemical reaction combined with new emotional material form new instinctive behaviors or habits.

Hypnotherapy starts with a meeting of the therapist and the client during which the hypnotherapist gets to know the client, learning something of his or her history, and developing rapport and communication. Identifying the behaviors that need attention is essential. Sometimes there may be a discussion regarding origins of the base behaviors, but hypnotherapy is mostly focused on changing future behavior from the current behavior. Often the events that generated the behaviors in the first place need not be addressed. Certain behaviors do require overcoming root causes, but more often than not, such steps are unnecessary. Once the broad first behaviors that set the stage for drug abuse are identified, the hypnotherapist and the client will establish goals for the therapy plan to change those underlying behaviors.

The second step is to identify habits associated with the actual drug abuse itself. These triggers can lead to the actions that foster the drug use, bringing on actual physical demand for drugs. These are behaviors that are identified with the act of taking a pill, using a hypodermic needle, or inhaling a substance. We are talking about a similar behavior when smokers have to have that cigarette with their first cups of coffee. What triggers lie at the heart of the substance abuser's activities? The therapist wants to identify those behaviors and develop ways for the client to avoid, overcome, or re-direct those behaviors.

Once a plan is developed, the therapist will utilize hypnosis to access the Middle Mind where the behaviors are locked in. Here, the hypnotherapy process is fascinating. Utilizing information obtained during the initial interview of the session, the therapist will form verbal suggestions to give to the client while he or she is in a state of hypnosis. In time, the client's very own subconscious will take these words and use them to overwrite the bad programming creating the destructive behaviors, developing new behaviors that simply take the place and control of the prior behaviors.

After the hypnosis session, the client, with practical directions in addition to the suggestions made during hypnosis, will then test his or her progress through real-world living and decision-making. Follow-up sessions will allow the client and hypnotherapist to evaluate progress and continuously improve and strengthen the client's new behaviors. In time, the new behaviors will become absolutely controlling and permanent. In this way, hypnotherapy proves itself as an effective and efficient method for overcoming drug abuse.

CHAPTER 35

VIDEO GAME ADDICTION (GAMING DISORDER)

More and more people are seeking help to deal with the psychological problems emerging from technology. One of these serious problems involves the addiction to video games. Youngsters are becoming addicted, but now we are seeing the phenomenon continue on into adulthood, particularly among Millennials. Many people use video games simply for entertainment and relaxation. Those who use games in order to relax at the end of the day are not necessarily addicted. However, for the addict, gaming hijacks the mind, and the qualities of addiction that we see with drugs and alcohol begin to manifest themselves with these individuals. The problem has become so severe that the World Health Organization has recognized the problem and named it. It is called Gaming Disorder.

Gaming Disorder is present when a player becomes compelled to play video games and requires constantly increasing engagement playing video games to achieve the same satisfaction or rush of pleasure. The playing of the video game is constantly on addicts' minds, so that they are visualizing the thrill of playing, advancing, improving, and enjoying the game, even when they are not playing. Addicts are always thinking about the next game. There exists always a desire to upgrade equipment and purchase new games. New games have different themes, newer graphics, and more advanced technology, and addicts are unconsciously compelled to spend money to acquire these new advances, followed by extraordinary amounts of time to advance their skills and knowledge with the new games. Suppliers of games and manufacturers of new technology are all too happy to take the addicts' money.

Beyond physical changes to the addict's mind, which are still being studied, video game addiction creates a number of social problems. For the students, grades are impacted as class or study time falls prey to gaming. For older players in the workforce, the ability to acquire and hold employment is compromised as gaming supersedes sleep and work. Social relationships for those with gaming disorder are strained, and video game players become isolated from their social circles. Often, video game addicts spend countless hours before their gaming systems, ultimately developing personal hygiene issues and sleep disorders.

Hypnotherapy offers effective and efficient relief from those suffering from Gaming Disorder. Of course, as with any addiction, individuals suffering with the problem need to have some level of desire to overcome their addictions. In a typical teenager, this desire may not be present since they may not fully recognize the impact of the addiction. It may be that a hypnotherapist, acting as an authoritative third party, can meet with a young person who does not desire to change. Such a meeting may help a young gamer to recognize the problems that gaming has created, and thus help to foster a desire for change. Once an addict desires a change, hypnotherapy can provide a solution.

At the heart of any addiction is a habit. This habit is a subconscious, Middle Mind act over which the individual has lost conscious control. This habit always wins out because the habit exists below consciousness, and since it lies within the Middle Mind, hypnosis provides the tool for the therapist to reach that habit. Once the Middle Mind is in play, the therapist can provide the client with the tools necessary to reprogram the habit. Speaking to the Middle Mind, the therapist will help the addict recognize the dangers associated with the addiction and help to create new, dominating aversions to gaming. The Middle Mind will focus on different, more effective behaviors. Clients will be given the tools to develop healthy life patterns and to establish conscious control over their behaviors. They will be provided with new skills to relax and build confidence. They will also learn steps to lessen anticipated withdrawal from the video gaming, such as irritability, depression, and compulsive thoughts. In the end, the goal of hypnotherapy will be empowering clients to set conscious priorities for their lives.

There must be no delay in addressing video gaming habits. We know that the video games and other technologies are starting to impact the brains of individuals. In video gamers, we are seeing the development of vision problems and posture problems. With ever-increasing technology and the marketing of technology targeting young people, getting control over the engagement with modern life cannot start too soon. Hypnotherapy offers real answers to this worsening problem.

CHAPTER 36

DIGITAL DEMENTIA & TECHNOLOGY ADDICTION

The numbers tell the story. On average, Americans today check their smartphones 52 times per day. For Millennials, that number skyrockets to 150 times per day. A recent study indicates that the average cell phone owner actually touches the phone in excess of 2600 times a day, with the most extreme phone users touching it over 5000 times a day. Smart phones on average are checked every 10 minutes. Baby Boomers spend five hours each day on their smartphone, and Millennials are on their phones nearly six hours each day. Thirteen percent of Millennials and five percent of Baby Boomers say they spend, get this, twelve hours every day on their phones. And that is just phone usage. Those numbers do not even include time spent on desktop computers, laptops, or tablets. In a sense, we could say that all people in today's world have some sort of addiction to technology. We are just beginning to understand how we may be physically damaging ourselves with all the technology connectedness that invades our everyday lives. We know that attention spans have dropped from 12 seconds to 8 seconds in the last few years, and we know that memory ability is diminished as we rely more and more on our devices.

Most of us have probably sensed at one time or another that we need to cut back on a technology. Those senior moments that many of us experience, such as forgetting why we walked into a room, or not being able to recall something that we know we know, are actually occurring more often and earlier, and that memory loss is now being connected to technology use. Digital dementia is characterized by deterioration of brain function as a result of overuse of technology. This overuse of technology causes a breakdown of cognitive ability, a loss of memory, and damage to vision. Increased anxiety and tension-related problems are also associated with technology use. The medical field tells us that structural changes occur through the overuse of technology, including the development of a problem informally known as "tech neck." We now have confirmed the development of more and various psychological disorders as a result of playing video games (See CHAPTER 35), and surely in time we are going to connect more physical and mental abnormalities to uses of technology.

It is ironic that developers of so much technology have been the first to realize the danger that is associated with overuse of technology. They now warn us about children being exposed to technology too early for fear of damage to their brain development, as well as the impact that technology may on the Middle Mind. Silicone Valley moguls themselves keep their children away from technology and send their children to schools that avoid using technology at all during the formative years.

Granted, technology is amazing. We now have access to an amazing amount of information that can be helpful in our daily lives. I certainly use technology for business-related purposes, for outside interests, and for social purposes. But I too have found myself at times disappointed in my own behavior when it comes to technology. It really hit home for me one day in a grocery store. As I was going down one aisle of the grocery store on a weekend morning, I checked my phone to see if I had any notifications or anything I needed to tend to. As I made my way to the next aisle, I found myself instinctively reaching from my phone and checking it again, on a day and at a time I knew there would be very little internet traffic. I resolved right then that I needed to temper my use. (I suspect my wife would still say I spend too much time connected.)

I assume that my issues are very moderate when I see the numbers that we set out above. But for those who are being wrapped up by technology and want to make a change, hypnotherapy provides a good starting point for gaining control over the addiction. As we have indicated in other chapters dealing with various forms of addiction, addictions are habits. Sometimes there is a chemical dependency, as with drug usage and alcoholism, which needs to be addressed. But other addictions are purely Middle Mind, subconscious behaviors. Technology usage has simply become instinctive for addicts. They do not think about its use, and they begrudge the times in which they cannot go online. Technology is destroying

261

some people as the habit becomes an outright need, sometimes superseding the needs of their own families, bodies, or lives. The behavior is totally non-thinking. When addicts who are physically and emotionally damaging themselves come to a point in which they realize that they need to make a change, they should explore hypnotherapy.

The goal of hypnotherapy is simple, but getting there varies from person to person. Since the technology addiction is a habit, we know it is unthinking behavior. When behavior is unthinking, it is originating in the Middle Mind or the subconscious (see CHAPTER 7), and it overwhelms and overrides an individual's thought processes. The overall goal of hypnotherapy will be to take this automatic, uncontrolled behavior and move it into the consciousness, so that clients can take back control of their behavior. One of the first goals of therapy is to change behavior so that clients recognize consciously what they are doing. The clients are no longer acting simply on instinct without being alerted in their conscious mind as to their behaviors. Recognition is a good starting point, but once the conscious mind realizes the behavior, is it going to make better decisions? Everybody has had the experience of being faced with a particular food that he knows he should not eat, but he eats it anyway. Similarly there needs to be strengthening of confidence and commitment to making right technology decisions for each tech-addicted client. These goals can be achieved with hypnotherapy, utilizing hypnosis.

Hypnosis is simply the bridge to the Middle Mind. It is not magic; it is a tool. Accessing the Middle Mind will not change anything. The work is what happens after a client is in hypnosis with the trained assistance of the hypnotherapist. Hypnosis is a safe activity in which the subject is well aware of everything that is taking place. The goal is simply to allow a client's own mind to resolve the issues. Hypnosis provides the mechanism to give the client the raw materials to make changes. These raw materials come in the form of suggestions, the term given to the verbal instructions the therapist uses during the process. Therapists and clients develop these suggestions during the pre-hypnosis stage of each session, so they are tailor-made for the particular needs of the client. Once the suggestions are received, a client's own mind will begin to reprogram itself. With the technology addict, the client will begin not only to recognize automatic behaviors, but also to gain control of them, and to make important behavior changes, confidently and instinctively. Hypnotherapy becomes the method to ending the madness.

CHAPTER 37

ANGER MANAGEMENT

How can you tell if anger is out of control? A number of signs may indicate a person needs help: if the anger has led to being charged with a crime, if it has led to violence against a partner, family member or others; if it leads to property damage; if it leads to regular arguments with others or constant feelings of anger; if there is a sense of loss of control because of anger, or if there is worry about what may happen because of anger. Hypnotherapy offers fast and effective tools for the person who needs help with anger management.

Anger, in and of itself, is not the problem. The problem lies with the person who cannot manage or control that behavior. People who experience any of the behaviors listed above probably have serious anger management problems that interfere with their personal and social lives. As with so many of our behaviors, these do not originate in the conscious, rational mind. These behaviors are instinctive habits and drives which have become super controllers of behavior not easily changed.

Those who cannot control anger can suffer serious long-term emotional and physical harm. Broken relationships, loss of jobs, and danger of physical harm to oneself or to others are frequent concerns. People with anger management problems may sabotage their own work, escape into silence, or lash out in sarcasm. It is important to get anger under control to successfully function in society.

Causes for anger management problems are varied and numerous. These destructive behaviors may be modeled behaviors that a child witnessed in his or her parents or others of influence. They may result from some form of frustration or powerlessness experienced during developmental years. Whatever the specific cause, the anger most likely developed from some actual situation that included strong emotions. A mature understanding of the situation may have prevented the behavior from being formed, but children often misinterpret or misunderstand situations. As a result, programming of the Middle Mind becomes corrupted.

In hypnotherapy, the therapist and the client will want to get some general sense of the causes of the anger issues, but only to identify whether or not there needs to be specific therapy directed to those causes. The goal of hypnotherapy will be to generate new thought patterns and avoid the negative thoughts that have led to the intense anger. One primary goal will be to identify and address triggers or different circumstances that may lead to either angry outbursts or continuing feelings of anger. Once those triggers are identified, therapy works to create a conscious awareness of when these events occur and to develop techniques to diffuse anger before it does harm. Therapy will help to create a confident calmness in the client and to give her the tools needed to relax. Hypnotherapy will also provide methods to deal with the side effects of continuing anger problems such as anxiety, depression, and stress.

A goal in therapy for the anger management client is the development of confidence in life that will allow a client to instantly identify situations or people that trigger angry behavior. It may be that certain words or attitudes set off the angry response. It could be that such behavior is generated by lack of exercise, or diet, or other physical or chemical factors. If so, an awareness and a plan to deal with those problems will be adopted. First, anger management clients need to develop clear objective views of the nature of their behaviors, grasping how those behavior are viewed by others. They must learn to step back from those triggering situations, to take deep breaths, and to remain calm. They also need to develop techniques for conversing rationally with others about matters of importance that previously had led to angry outbursts or angry feelings.

Hypnosis is simply a tool that hypnotherapists use to reach a client's Middle Mind. The therapy includes not only the hypnosis, but the total engagement between the therapist and the client. This engagement includes the background development, the therapeutic planning process, and the practical follow up to each hypnotherapy session. From session one, the client should start to see the impact of the therapeutic process. The exact number of sessions will be established early, usually during the first session. With each successive session, progress will be evaluated, and more steps to permanent behavior change implemented.

Hypnotherapy is an effective means for permanently

changing anger problems. Because of the long-term damage that a lack of anger management can create, people who struggle with their anger should seize the opportunity to undergo hypnotherapy as soon as possible.

CHAPTER 38

DEPRESSION

I once heard someone describe depression as feeling "like I had no past and no future." In a very general sense, depression describes a wide variety of emotions and physical responses or behaviors. Since these are destructive emotions or behaviors, we can conclude that they originate in the Middle Mind or the subconscious. As a result, hypnotherapy offers successful, non-pharmaceutical means of coping with and overcoming depression.

Depression has a number of indicators: persistent feelings of sadness, despondency, emptiness, or hopelessness. Many experience periods of angry outbursts. Typically, the depressed person loses interest in things that normally would cause pleasure, such as engaging in a hobby, eating a favorite meal, or enjoying romantic activities. Various forms of sleep disorders, such as insomnia, often accompany depression. A depressed person typically feels tired and lifeless, lacking energy. Sufferers may experience a lack of appetite and weight loss, or conversely, constant food cravings and weight gain.

Some may experience heightened anxiety and restlessness. Everything seems to be in slow motion to the depressed person, from thinking to physical movements. They may experience trouble with focus, and in severe cases, they may have recurrent thoughts of death and suicide. Continued depression can eventually lead to physical problems that will exacerbate the depression.

None of us can escape someEveryone experiences some episodes of depression in their lives. The death of a loved one, going through a divorce, or even something like moving can cause periods of depression as life's routines are disturbed, questions about life and existence impinge upon our daily lives, or we are confronted with a physical injury or other health issue. These forms of depression can be alleviated in hypnotherapy, but this chapter deals primarily with the long-term persistent depression that begins to impact relationships, employment, school, and more.

The Middle Mind or subconscious holds the key to depression since we know that we cannot simply rationalize our way out of those overwhelming emotions. Some programming of the subconscious is contributing to these various symptoms; therefore, we know that improvement can occur through hypnotherapy. A simple scan through the table of contents of this book shows that hypnotherapy can address nearly every manifestation of depression. Therefore, if we have an accumulated bundle of these symptoms, treatment through hypnotherapy can be used to unpack and address each condition. In many cases, the depression is not the cause of the symptom, but rather the identified symptom is actually the cause of the depression. For instance, a person suffering from a sleep disorder like insomnia will over time begin to experience elements of depression, from despondency to tiredness to anger. The person who is well overweight is persistently hit with clothes that fit too tightly, photographs that disappoint, and the lack of pleasure in a number of otherwise enjoyable activities. Overweight people always have some element of depression, some more than others. Depression can eventually become so serious, adversely impacting so many areas, that sufferers contemplate self-harm or suicide.

Before going for medically prescribed antidepressants, those experiencing depression need to see a hypnotherapist. Within hypnotherapy sessions, therapists will seek to understand the depressed client, unearth all the symptoms, and explore all the possible causes. As the cornerstone of the therapy, hypnosis is used to find the base issues that are making it impossible for the clients to "think" their way out of the condition. As with most hypnotherapy, there will be a focus on helping clients learn to automatically relax and avoid the stresses of their condition. Therapists will also seek to strengthen clients' confidence and create positive self-views. With the ability to break down the various elements of the depression, the causes and the responses, therapists can help clients see their circumstances more objectively, understand what they are dealing with, and change their behavioral responses. The transformation can be quick, leading to long-term, permanent changes.

Because hypnotherapy offers such a broad application to a client's needs, it is something that certainly should be considered by any person grappling with symptoms of depression.

CHAPTER 39

TINNITUS

Millions of people are affected by tinnitus, a perception of ringing, clicking, buzzing, or hissing sounds in the ear. Subjective tinnitus describes a condition in which sufferers perceive the noise internally without having an actual physical cause for the noise. Those suffering from subjective tinnitus have found hypnotherapy effective in alleviating their symptoms.

There are forms of tinnitus that do have physical causes. Therefore, before a hypnotherapist will treat a client with tinnitus, that client will need medical testing in order to rule out a physical cause. The physical causes that lead to tinnitus may include ear infections, wax build-up, high blood pressure, thyroid problems, or diabetes. Once it is determined that there is no physical cause for the ringing or clicking, then hypnotherapy becomes a viable and recognized treatment for the condition.

Hypnotherapy for tinnitus is one example of the absolute value of hypnosis-based, Middle Mind therapy. Once possible physical causes are eliminated, a sufferer needs no further search for the cause of the problem. Hypnotherapy will create an ability to live without the frustrations associated with the continuous ringing in the ears. For some people, that ringing in the ears is sporadic, while for others it is constant. For those who have the serious forms of tinnitus, the continuous noise can create mental and emotional challenges, ultimately leading to physical problems, as well. Getting the tinnitus under control can improve a sufferer's daily life immensely.

Subjective tinnitus is very individualistic; each client has distinctive problems and personal impacts on daily living. The hypnotherapist wants to get to know the specifics of the client's condition and tailor the hypnotherapy sessions to that particular client. The ultimate goal of the hypnotherapy is to push the irritating noises deep into the background of the client's consciousness so that the mind no longer takes note of the irritating sounds. The Middle Mind will simply ignore the unwanted sounds, avoiding the constant impact to the client's life. The client's reaction to the sounds will change, so that the client will no longer live dreading its return. Hypnotherapy does not cure the tinnitus, but it does allow the individual to overcome it.

One typical step in the hypnotherapy treatment of tinnitus is to train the client in the use of self-hypnosis, a tool that the client will be able to use to relax and cope with the condition. The self-hypnosis will work as a reinforcement to the hypnotherapy, providing a more permanent resolution to the problem.

If you or a loved one is suffering with subjective tinnitus, consider seeking relief through hypnotherapy, which has repeatedly proven effective in providing the necessary tools to cope with the condition. Tinnitus should no longer be a constant, cruel interruption in anyone's life!

CHAPTER 40

MIGRAINES

Some twelve percent of Americans suffer with migraines, a debilitating and recurring type of headache. Women suffer with migraines with three times the frequency as men. Often, a migraine is painful on only one side of the head and is accompanied by nausea, weakness, and severe sensitivity to light, sounds, and odors. People who suffer from migraines often have a family history of the condition. Medical, physical, or environmental factors may also lead to migraines, such as epilepsy, certain types of medicine, tobacco usage, caffeine intake, hormone changes, medication overuse, food additives, and over-exertion. However, because a number of behavioral causes exists, hypnotherapy offers an effective treatment to lessen or eliminate migraine pain.

Behavioral factors precipitating migraines include stress, anxiety, depression, sleep disorders, diet, bodily reactions to changes in the weather, and responses to bright lights, loud sounds or strong smells. Many of these particular causes are addressed in other chapters of Part III. Hypnotherapy can resolve these particular causes directly, thereby lessening or totally eliminating migraines. Studies have repeatedly shown that hypnotherapy is much more successful in treating migraines than medication, and, of course, it comes without the concerns associated with the side effects of drugs.

Often, a person who regularly experiences migraines can anticipate when one is approaching. The first stage in the migraine headache process is known as the *prodome*, which happens within the preceding twenty-four hours before the onset of the full headache. Some characteristics of the prodome are food cravings, mood changes, and yawning. The second stage of the migraine, the *aura*, occurs just before or during the migraine. During the aura, migraine sufferers may experience flashing or bright lights or zig-zag lines in their vision. They may become physically weaker and highly sensitive to touch.

Stage three is the headache itself, characterized by throbbing pain, nausea or vomiting, and increased sensitivity to light, sounds, and odors. Sometimes the migraine actually exists without a headache, but for most, the headache is one of the worst parts. In stage four, or the *postdrome*, the pain has passed, but the sufferer is left exhausted, weak, and confused. The postdrome can last up to a full day.

Migraine headaches can be debilitating, and often those who suffer regularly with migraines live not only in fear and anticipation, but also in the worry of the interruption to normal life that accompanies pain and other challenges of a migraine.

Hypnotherapy is very effective in rapidly addressing conditions that cause migraines, providing tools to the individual to lessen or eliminate migraines altogether. In one case study, a woman had suffered migraines for fifteen years. In eight sessions her condition was greatly improved, and ten months later she reported that she was no longer experiencing migraines. Using self-hypnosis, she was able to continue her success after therapy sessions had ended.

Before hypnotherapy will begin, therapist will first confirm what, if any, physical causes are creating the condition. No therapist wants to take steps that mask a serious problem. Once the sessions begin, the hypnotherapist works to gain an understanding of the behavioral factors that may be contributing to the onset of migraines. With the client, the therapist will develop plans to address these factors as part of the therapy. The therapy will include hypnosis, which allows mastery of the problems at the Middle Mind, or subconscious, level. The therapist will use specialized techniques to help the client better relax and respond preemptively to the onset of a migraine.

Since many sufferers have the advantage of sensing its onset, hypnotherapists can offer tools to help them avoid the migraine all together. The hypnotherapist can also train the client in self-hypnosis to apply and reinforce the gains made during the original hypnotherapy. Applying self-hypnosis is effective not only for adults, but also for children and adolescents who suffer with migraines. Many times, migraines can be completely avoided, but even if a migraine starts, hypnotherapy offers effective tools to lessen the pain and diminish the other issues that come with the headache. As with all hypnotherapy, the goal is that all progress will remain permanent. Whether or not a person has recently started having migraines or has been suffering with them for years, there is no time like the present to get relief. And that relief comes with hypnosis-based therapy.

CHAPTER 41

ASTHMA

Asthma is a chronic respiratory disease affecting many Americans. The American Lung Association estimates that six million children under the age of eighteen suffer from asthma. Asthma has no known specific causes, but studies suggest some combination of heredity and environmental factors bring on the disease. Asthma has physiological causes, and a medical doctor should always be consulted prior to the involvement of a hypnotherapist. However, hypnotherapy has proven to be a valuable benefit to those suffering with asthma.

Asthma is a breathing disorder often characterized by shallow breathing, uncontrollable coughing, wheezing, shortness of breath, chest tightening, and sleep difficulties. The airways of the asthma sufferer are obstructed and can become inflamed. Whether brought about by physical triggers such as allergies, work environments, and exercise, or psychological triggers, such as stress and anxiety, hypnosis-based therapy can provide relief from asthma. For those psychological triggers, hypnotherapy can even help to prevent an asthmatic attack.

Those who suffer with asthma often demonstrate some level of high anxiety, high dependence on others, low confidence, or suppressed emotions. All of these behaviors are some form of Middle Mind, or subconscious, behaviors that hypnotherapy can address.

Certain events can instinctively generate serious fear, fright, and panic in all of us. Not being able to breathe would certainly be high on the list of natural fears. As a result, when an asthma attack occurs, it is natural to panic. Unfortunately, this overly emotional response makes everything worse. As attacks happen, the fear in the anticipation of the next attack actually contributes to more attacks. As attacks occur, the circumstances surrounding the attacks become embedded in the subconscious, so that when the asthma sufferer confronts similar circumstances, the attacks are triggered. This psychological conditioning, known to some as the law of unintended consequences, actually works against the asthma sufferer: the more the sufferer seeks to avoid a particular result (the asthma), the more frequently that unintended result occurs (the asthma).

Hypnotherapy can first address the asthma client's overall behavioral makeup. If general anxiety, stress, depression, or lack of confidence exists and is contributing to the ailment, hypnotherapy can identify the issues and deal with them. If other emotions are being unnecessarily suppressed and that suppression leads to attacks, a plan for overcoming this trigger can be developed. Because so much of an asthma attack is triggered by stress, with another level of stress occurring during the attack, the client learns to relax before the attack occurs and then to avoid the panic and stress through relaxation during an attack. This relaxation will lessen the effects of an attack and end it quicker. Because hypnosis is the key to reaching some of the embedded drives and instincts that are contributing to the initiation of attacks and the severity of attacks, hypnotherapy will include periods of hypnosis in a typical session. The asthma client will learn particular relaxation techniques, often including self-hypnosis, that will become tools for coping more successfully with asthma.

Studies show that hypnotherapy is valuable in helping asthma sufferers overcome those debilitating effects of asthma. No child or adult need deal with overwhelming effects of asthma as often or as severely as they are presently. Get help now.

CHAPTER 42

CONFIDENCE & SELF-ESTEEM

T he prevalence of low confidence and low self-esteem is evident in the self-help section of any bookstore. Unfortunately, the effectiveness of the books depends upon our ability to talk ourselves into more confidence and higher esteems, a method that many people find difficult to accomplish. Hypnotherapy, however, is quite effective as treatment for both these issues. On the surface, these may seem to be related problems, but they are distinguishable. While they are very personal and distinctive to each individual client, the causes, manifestations of the conditions, and impacts upon each client's life are all very individualistic. Therefore, treatments will involve a thorough examination specific to each client.

Let's define and distinguish the ideas of confidence and self-esteem. Confidence deals with specific abilities or qualities in one's life. Self-esteem, though, is more of an overall sense or feeling about oneself. One who is low on confidence lacks self-assurance in a personal ability or quality. One who is low in self-esteem has a low overall feeling of self-worth or self-value. An individual may have an overall positive self-value, but may lack confidence in specific areas. For example, a high school student may be a star athlete on the field or court, but that student may suffer greatly in confidence when asked to read out loud, give a speech, or take a test. She may not lack the intellectual skills to perform well; she is simply lacking in confidence. The individual dealing with low self-esteem is generally impacted, to some extent, in all areas of life because she feels unworthy.

Confidence and self-esteem also impact lives in different ways. Lack of confidence stunts personal development. For instance, with our athlete example, although she may excel in sports and reap the rewards, she is limited by poor grades or by avoiding opportunities she may otherwise have. Ultimately, it might limit her choice of avocations. Of course, every one of these lost opportunities or avoided activities will impact her personal development. Low self-esteem can have an even more pervasive and damaging effect upon an individual. Since low self-esteem is considered a personality trait, it becomes practically a permanent aspect of a person's entire life. Thinking poorly of themselves, they may become socially reclusive, become depressed, develop social phobias, and even turn to alcohol or drugs to mask their insecurities.

The causes of these conditions may start fairly early. Events and relationships during early developmental stages may be the cause, or, as happens in so many cases with confidence and self-esteem issues, relationships and events during those early critical years in school will lead to a lack of confidence and self esteem. A therapist will determine early in the hypnotherapy sessions whether or not the exploration of causes is necessary. Generally, hypnotherapy is a forward-looking exercise. In other words, regardless of the cause of the lack of confidence or the low self-esteem, hypnotherapy will deal with future behaviors and feelings. However, having at least a general sense of the facts that initiated the conditions will be important.

The hypnotherapist will also be interested in the daily impact the low confidence or poor self-worth is having in the client's life. These facts are important because the therapist is always concerned with producing practical and immediate impacts on daily activities and attitudes. Once an inventory is taken of these various causes and manifestations of the condition, the hypnotherapist will work with a client to develop a plan that will be used both during the sessions of hypnosis and in real-world applications. As part of the hypnotherapy sessions, the client will spend short periods of time in hypnosis, time in which the plan will be implemented. This implementation involves taking the specific goals established in the therapeutic plan, and providing them to the client's Middle Mind, or subconscious, in such a way that the client's mind, the hero of every hypnotherapy story, goes to work doing a mental makeover. The hypnotherapist will take steps to strengthen the ego of the client in order to increase his optimism, coping skills, energy, and positive self-talk.

When I was first introduced to hypnotherapy as a client for weight loss, my hypnotherapist helped me develop anchors for confidence that I use to this day, not only when dealing with eating issues, but also as I deal with other areas of life. With low confidence or low self-esteem, using anchors will give the client valuable tools for daily living.

One of the exciting elements for hypnotherapists who work with clients suffering from low self-confidence or diminished self-esteem is knowing that these clients will have futures that includes more joy and personal growth. Hypnotherapy changes lives.

CHAPTER 43

OBSESSIVE THOUGHTS

For those having trouble with obsessive thoughts - ideas, images, or words that are constantly intruding upon one's thought - hypnotherapy provides relief. Because these thoughts are unwanted and uncontrollable, ultimately, they impact a person's life, sapping enjoyment and replacing it with worry and anxiety.

The reason that hypnotherapy works is that it provides the key for persons to control the uncontrollable of their minds. It is not that behavior is permanently uncontrollable; it is just that part of the mind, the Middle Mind, is not controlled by thinking, logical, or conscious activity. When we are faced with such uncontrollable behaviors, we are dealing with issues within the Middle Mind, more frequently called the subconscious. This subconscious houses many functions that are essential to life. Here lie not only the operations of our bodily functions, but also the many positive instincts and habits essential for day-to-day life.

However, from time to time, behaviors can get programmed

in the Middle Mind that we would love to change, but we do not know how. For some, it may be overeating, nail biting, or some other "unconscious" activity. For those suffering with obsessive thoughts, the Middle Mind is generating intrusive thoughts that interfere with daily life. The first benefit of hypnotherapy is giving a person suffering with obsessive thoughts access to the cause of the issue in the Middle Mind. Once she has a strong understanding of her client, a trained hypnotherapist can help that client develop an individualized game plan to use in taking back control of his thoughts consciously. Then, utilizing hypnosis, which is the key to unlocking access to the Middle Mind, the hypnotherapist will lead the client to the place where the problem exists. Using their plan, the therapist provides the suggestions to the client's Middle Mind, the raw materials necessary for changes to be made. Then, the client's own Middle Mind takes over and does its magic, reprogramming the troubling behavior.

With obsessive thoughts, the goal is to move control over this portion of the thought life from the subconscious into the thinking, conscious mind. Once this move is accomplished, the client can sort through the thoughts calmly and dispassionately, reassigning the disturbing thoughts to a category of lesser importance. Being able to objectively deal with the thoughts at the conscious level gives the client the ability to eliminate the uncontrolled intrusion of the thoughts in daily life. Gaining control over one's thought life offers people a new level of confidence and happiness.

CHAPTER 44

BEREAVEMENT & CHRONIC GRIEF

T
o grieve is a normal experience. With the death of a loved one, an individual can experience a full range of emotions that can last from days to years. Bereavement that needs some form of intervention such as hypnotherapy may be characterized as complicated bereavement or chronic grief. If the duration of the grief extends beyond what most would consider as normal, then outside help may be necessary. If the intensity of the grief interferes with life and wellbeing, help may be necessary. Additionally, if bereavement manifests itself in identifiable emotional, psychological, and physical ways that do not promote well-being, help may be necessary.

Often, these serious forms of grief are connected to the nature of the death. Loss of life that was traumatic, totally unexpected, and/or sudden can trigger issues of chronic grief. Children of a parent who has died often experience lifetime emotional problems if the complicated bereavement is not addressed. The cause of these long-term, or chronic, problems is that the severe emotions are occurring in the individual's mind which is trying to interpret all the factual circumstances related to the death. All these thoughts and emotions overwhelm the conscious mind, and it is in the Middle Mind, or the subconscious, where these jumbled thoughts and emotions wrap together and solidify. Occasionally, the Middle Mind is not able to sort out all this information and intensity, and the resulting mental residue is undesired behaviors and debilitating emotional and physical responses. Hypnotherapy provides the key to getting at this distorted mental programming and reorganizing it in a more functional pattern.

People suffering from complicated bereavement or chronic grief take on a very pessimistic outlook on life. They may give up on goals and effort, become very negative about life events, or interpret all their day-to-day activities through a negative prism of grief. They may develop a great lack of trust in others. Some may become frantically active in meaningless activities, while others may be frozen and numb to life. Chronic grief may lead to sleep problems, such as nightmares, or simply a loss of ability to rest. Physical problems may begin to manifest themselves as chronic depression deepens. Such physical problems may become more serious health issues that doctors deem psychosomatic since they have ruled out any physical diagnosis of the causes. For instance, someone suffering this level of grief might develop fibromyalgia. In some cases, doctors may formally diagnose a sufferer with depression or anxiety disorder. It would not be unusual to see some addictive behavior developer or worsen as the grief continues.

Since these emotions and behaviors are uncontrolled, we know they originate in the Middle Mind. As a result, hypnotherapy provides the most beneficial response to the needs of the person grieving. The first step in therapy is to access the mis-programmed Middle Mind. Hypnosis is the key to opening the door to the subconscious. It is a safe and effective means of therapy with no side effects in which the grieving client is fully aware and in ultimate control of the process. In fact, it will be the client's Middle Mind which ultimately produces the desired results. Depending upon all the circumstances of the individual cases, the hypnotherapist might take several therapeutic routes. Typically, therapy includes some form of closure or dealing with unfinished business. One of the primary benefits with hypnosis is that it allows a client to deal with all the facts of the death again, but this time in a safe, organized, and objective fashion. With the swirl of emotions eliminated from the process, the client can look again at the event and all of its surrounding circumstances. This objective view allows the Middle Mind to reorganize all of these thoughts and to move them off center stage, so to speak. The grieving client can put the life of the lost one, with all the attendant history and relationship, back in order and within in a proper perspective. The client, now perhaps for the first time, can relax, return to an optimistic outlook, and rejoice in the memory of the one lost love one.

Death is a reality with which we all must deal, but sometimes reality can hit a person in such a way as to throw life a bit out of whack. Many people over time can naturally return to a state of normalcy, but for others, the sadness and grief become so debilitating and confused that a little assistance is needed. Living in such a dark place with chronic grief and bereavement does not have to imprison anyone now that we understand better how and why it occurs. Hypnotherapy provides the means to setting the mind in order and providing peace.